Basic Electrocardiography in Ten Days

David R. Ferry, MD

Chief, Cardiology Section
Jerry L. Pettis Memorial VA Medical Center
Associate Professor of Medicine
Loma Linda University School of Medicine

Foreword by Robert A. O'Rourke, MD

McGraw-Hill
Medical Publishing Division

NEW YORK   ST. LOUIS   SAN FRANCISCO   AUCKLAND
BOGOTÁ   CARACAS   LISBON   LONDON   MADRID
MEXICO CITY   MILAN   MONTREAL   NEW DELHI
SAN JUAN   SINGAPORE   SYDNEY   TOKYO   TORONTO

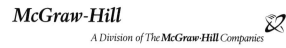

McGraw-Hill

A Division of The McGraw·Hill Companies

Basic Electrocardiography in Ten Days

1 2 3 4 5 6 7 8 9 0   QWKQWK   0 9 8 7 6 5 4 3 2 1 0

ISBN 0-07-135292-9

This book was set in Garamond by V&M Graphics, Inc.
The editors were Darlene B. Cooke, Kathleen McCullough, and Curt Berkowitz.
The production supervisor was Phil Galea.
The text designer was Patrice Sheridan.
The cover designer was Mary Skudlarek.

Quebecor World/Kingsport was the printer and binder.

This book is printed on acid-free paper.

This book is dedicated and written for

the medical students of Loma Linda University.

They were my inspiration and

my *de facto* editorial committee.

Table of Contents

Foreword

Dr. David Ferry, Associate Professor of Medicine from Loma Linda University, has produced an outstanding, user-friendly textbook utilizing computer-generated electrocardiograms for teaching electrocardiography in ten days. It is an excellent approach for medical students, nurses, physicians assistants, primary physicians, and cardiology trainees who wish to develop considerable expertise in the interpretation of abnormal electrocardiograms and in the proper identification of cardiac arrhythmias.

Dr. Ferry, who is a credit to our cardiology training program in San Antonio, has developed a very practical and successful method of teaching electrocardiography during the past two decades. As an effective teacher of electrocardiography to students at all levels, Dr. Ferry has developed outstanding illustrations of cardiac arrhythmias and ECG abnormalities such as ventricular hypertrophy and myocardial ischemia.

The computer-derived illustrations in this "ten day course" facilitate the learning of electrocardiography in a relaxed, nonstressful manner and the student can progress at his or her own pace in understanding ECGs and the interpretation of arrhythmias.

I am proud to recommend, with great enthusiasm, Dr. David Ferry's method for learning the basics of electrocardiography and obtaining the expertise to define abnormal electrocardiograms. Dr. Ferry has developed a superb teaching model that enables various members of the health care delivery system to learn electrocardiology and provide correct interpretation of the many abnormalities that can be diagnosed with this inexpensive, non-invasive technique.

Dr. Ferry is to be congratulated for his efforts.

Robert A. O'Rourke, MD, FACC, MACP
Charles Conrad Brown Distinguished Professorship in Cardiovascular Disease
Division of Cardiology
Department of Medicine
University of Texas Health Science Center at San Antonio

Preface

This book arose from our commitment to teach senior medical students how to interpret electrocardiograms in two weeks, or ten working days. The School of Medicine, in its wisdom, had chosen that interval for us, and we were forced to adapt to its mandate. We had 10 to 15 students in our class every four weeks for the entire academic year. We quickly realized that we needed to establish specific topics for each day so that, regardless of which faculty members were available, there was a consistent method used. We also decided on a set of sample ECGs to use each day.

I found myself repeatedly drawing the same illustrations, charts, and diagrams, so I eventually put together the rudiments of this text into a handout. This effort was well received by medical students, residents from Internal Medicine, Family Practice, and Preventive Medicine, and nurses and technicians. I was subsequently encouraged to publish this material, and the editors at McGraw-Hill were gracious enough to accommodate me.

All of the illustrations and electrocardiograms in this text were drawn on an Apple Macintosh G4 computer using Adobe Illustrator 8.0. Many of the drawings were drawn freehand in Illustrator, and others were drawn on paper, scanned into Adobe PhotoShop 5.5, transferred to Illustrator, and traced over. All of the ECGs were scanned into PhotoShop and traced over in Illustrator. The advantage of this technique is that all of the images and ECGs in this text are drawn (vector) images, which allows for the highest resolution at any magnification.

David R. Ferry, MD

Acknowledgments

I would like to thank my colleagues at the Jerry L. Pettis VAMC, Drs. Geir P. Frivold, Alan K. Jacobson, and Glenn L. Foster, for their constant suggestions and corrections. Many of the features of this text are the result of quiet, continuous gentle pressure applied by my friend Geir Frivold. The medical students made countless suggestions, found innumerable typos, and told me what worked and what didn't. My wife, Dr. Linda H. Ferry, was a reliable source of wisdom and inspiration. My editors at McGraw-Hill, Darlene Cooke and Kathleen McCullough, were invaluable. Finally, the encouragement of my mentor from my fellowship days, Dr. Robert A. O'Rourke, was very helpful and gratifying.

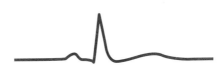

Suggestions for Using This Book

This book is arranged in a progressive manner, starting with basic concepts and increasing in complexity with the study of arrhythmias on Days 6, 7, and 8. The final two chapters cover miscellaneous topics and an introduction to electronic pacemakers. I suggest that the reader study the text and illustrations for each day in depth, and then interpret the electrocardiograms at the end of each chapter. The reader's interpretations should be compared with those appearing after the tracings. Although the information in this book is normally taught over a two week period to our students and residents, or over a few hours in seminars for practicing physicians, any amount of time necessary can be devoted by the reader. Day 6 in particular, because of its 30 ECGs may require a considerably greater effort. I recommend that the reader acquire sample ECGs from clinical sources and practice interpreting them.

Be systematic! Use the protocol suggested at the end of Day 1 and follow it rigorously. Using a system has two benefits: it forces the interpreter to be thorough and not overlook diagnoses, and it promotes organization of thought which will likely lead to a diagnosis.

Since this text represents the efforts of many collaborators and should be considered a work in progress, suggestions for future editions would be greatly appreciated. Please contact me at:

drferry@aol.com

Basic Electrocardiography in Ten Days

Day 1

The Basics

I. Components of the conduction system

A. The conduction system consists of modified cardiac muscle cells which
    have unique electrical properties.

B. Sinoatrial (SA) node
    1. The SA node is a tiny (1 mm) collection of cells in the upper right
        corner of the right atrium.
    2. The SA node controls the rhythm of the heart by virtue of having the
        fastest intrinsic rate of depolarization (60–100 beats/min).
    3. The SA node starts the cardiac cycle by initiating atrial systole.

C. The atrioventricular (AV) node
    1. The AV node is located near the inferior portion of the interatrial septum.
    2. The AV node serves two functions:
        a. It provides a physiological conduction delay to allow the atria to
            fill the ventricles prior to ventricular systole.
        b. It protects the ventricles from excessive stimulation from the atria,
            such as in atrial fibrillation.

D. The His-Purkinje system
    1. The His bundle divides into the right and left bundles.
    2. The left bundle further divides into the left anterior and posterior
        fascicles.
    3. The His-Purkinje system provides for the orderly depolarization of the
        ventricles.

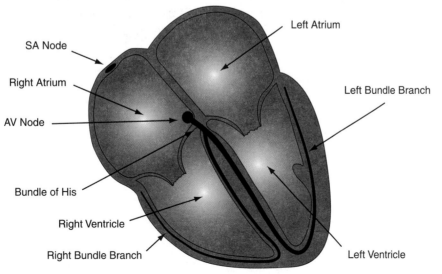

II. Genesis of the surface electrocardiogram

A. A wave of negative electrical potential spreads across the contracting myocardium.

B. This potential can be detected by electrodes placed at various locations on the skin and the signal amplified and displayed as an electrocardiogram (ECG).

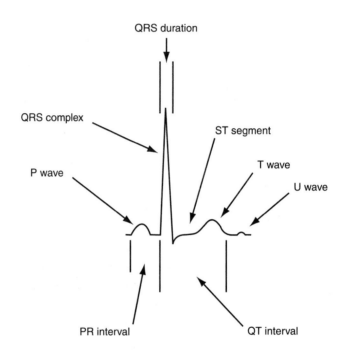

C. The components of the ECG represent various cardiac events
1. The P wave corresponds to atrial systole.
2. The PR interval represents the physiological delay in the AV node.
3. The QRS complex results from ventricular systole.
4. The T wave represents ventricular repolarization.

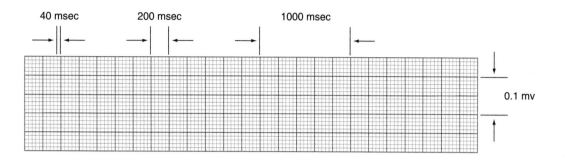

D. The ECG paper
  1. The ECG is recorded on moving paper ruled at 1 mm intervals with darker lines every 5 mm.
  2. At the standard paper speed of 25 mm/sec, each 1 mm horizontally represents 40 msec and each 5 mm interval 200 msec.
  3. In the vertical dimension, each 10 mm represents 0.1 mv of electrical potential.

III. The standard ECG leads

  A. There are six standard leads (the "limb leads") which depict cardiac electrical events from six angles in the frontal or vertical plane.

  B. There are six standard leads (the "chest leads") which depict electrical events in the horizontal plane.

ELECTROCARDIOGRAPHIC LEADS

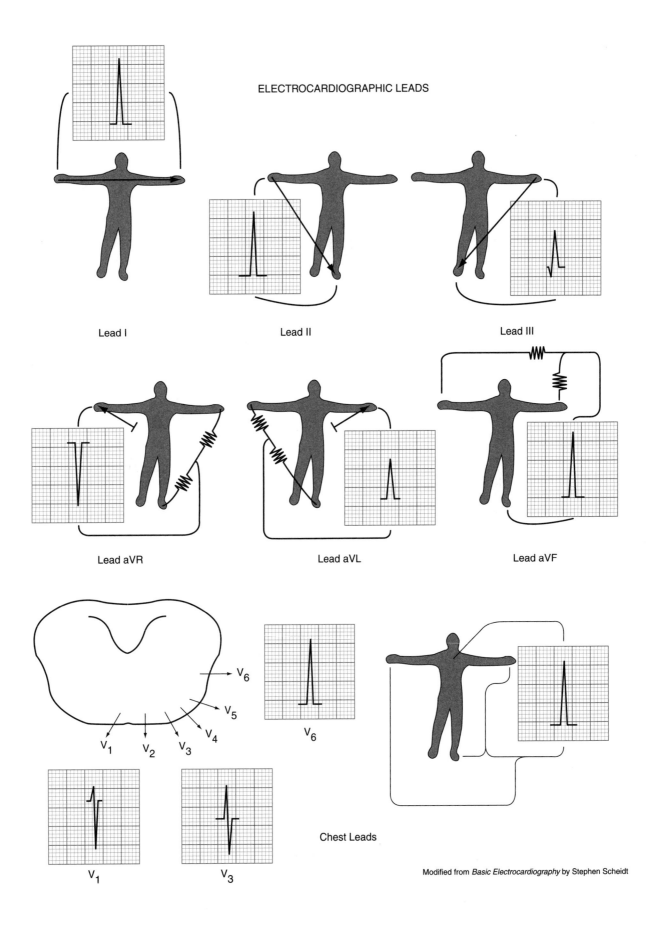

Lead I   Lead II   Lead III

Lead aVR   Lead aVL   Lead aVF

V_1 V_2 V_3 V_4 V_5 V_6

V_6

V_1 V_3

Chest Leads

Modified from *Basic Electrocardiography* by Stephen Scheidt

IV. Genesis of the ECG wave forms in the various leads and the concept of axis

    A. The P wave, QRS complex, and T wave for any lead can be derived from the vector representation of electrical activity in the appropriate plane.

        1. For instance, ventricular depolarization in the frontal plane can be displayed by a series of vectors representing the mathematical sum of all the electrical activity occurring at that instant.

        2. The origin of the vectors is in the left ventricle because most of the muscle mass is in that chamber.

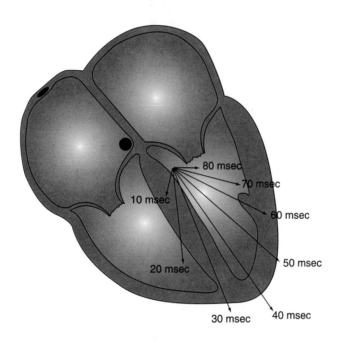

        3. The tips of these vectors can be connected to form a loop.

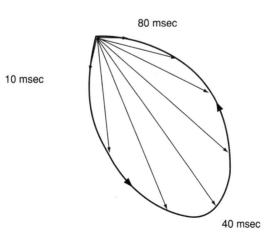

4. The loop can be superimposed on the frontal plane axis.

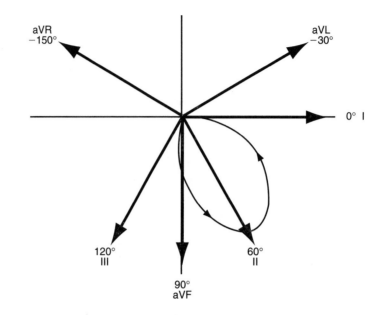

a. To form the QRS complex of Lead I, a line is drawn perpendicular to that lead.
b. By convention, all electrical forces on the side of the perpendicular towards Lead I are designated as positive, and those away as negative.

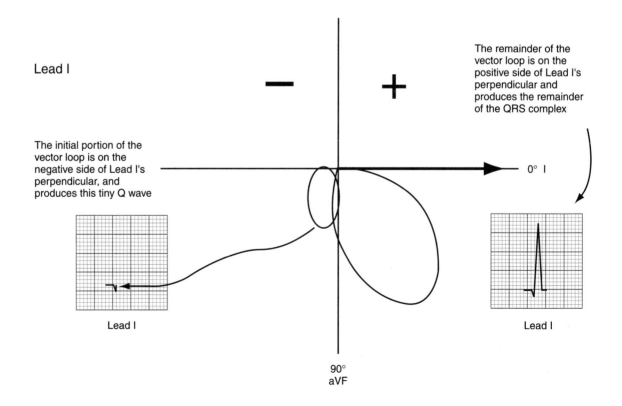

Lead aVF

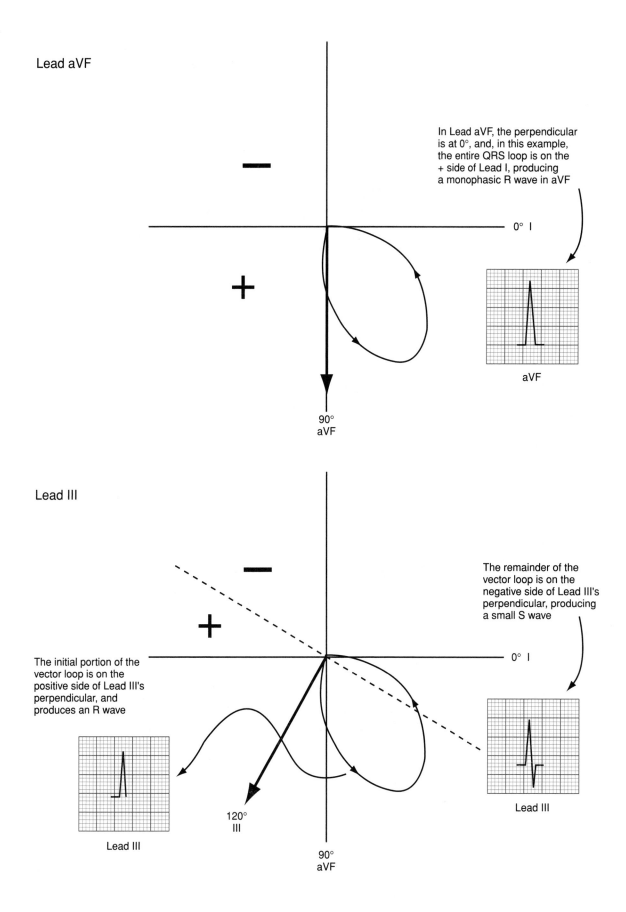

In Lead aVF, the perpendicular is at 0°, and, in this example, the entire QRS loop is on the + side of Lead I, producing a monophasic R wave in aVF

0° I

aVF

90°
aVF

Lead III

The remainder of the vector loop is on the negative side of Lead III's perpendicular, producing a small S wave

0° I

The initial portion of the vector loop is on the positive side of Lead III's perpendicular, and produces an R wave

Lead III

120°
III

Lead III

90°
aVF

B. The electrical axis is the sum of all the vectors in that plane
    1. The normal QRS axis is between −30° and +90°.

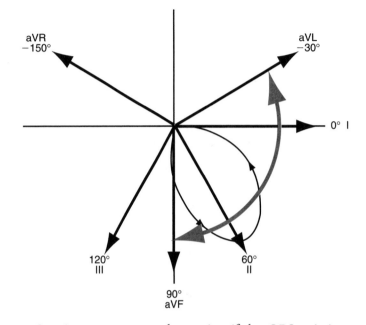

2. An easy way to determine if the QRS axis is normal is to examine
    Leads I and aVF, and, if necessary, Lead II.

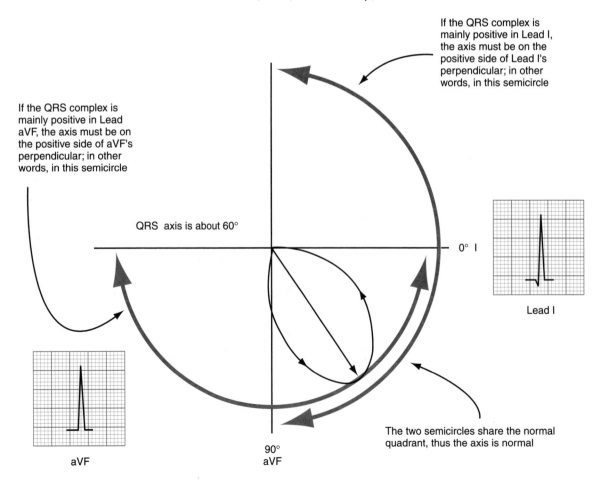

If the QRS complex is mainly positive in Lead I, the axis must be on the positive side of Lead I's perpendicular; in other words, in this semicircle

If the QRS complex is mainly positive in Lead aVF, the axis must be on the positive side of aVF's perpendicular; in other words, in this semicircle

QRS axis is about 60°

The two semicircles share the normal quadrant, thus the axis is normal

Lead I

aVF

0° I

90°
aVF

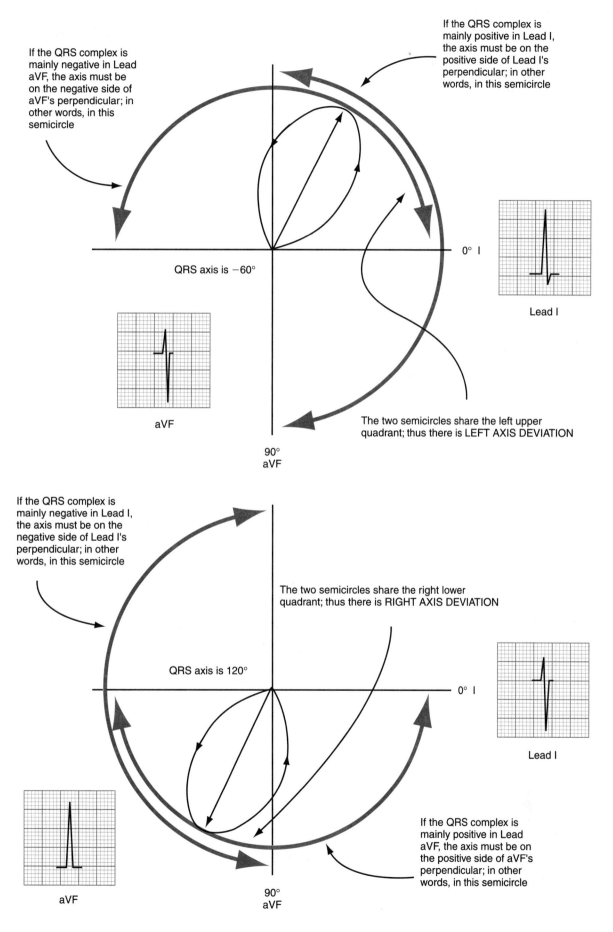

If the QRS complex is mainly negative in Lead aVF, the axis must be on the negative side of aVF's perpendicular; in other words, in this semicircle

If the QRS complex is mainly positive in Lead I, the axis must be on the positive side of Lead I's perpendicular; in other words, in this semicircle

QRS axis is −60°

0° I

Lead I

aVF

The two semicircles share the left upper quadrant; thus there is LEFT AXIS DEVIATION

90°
aVF

If the QRS complex is mainly negative in Lead I, the axis must be on the negative side of Lead I's perpendicular; in other words, in this semicircle

The two semicircles share the right lower quadrant; thus there is RIGHT AXIS DEVIATION

QRS axis is 120°

0° I

Lead I

aVF

If the QRS complex is mainly positive in Lead aVF, the axis must be on the positive side of aVF's perpendicular; in other words, in this semicircle

90°
aVF

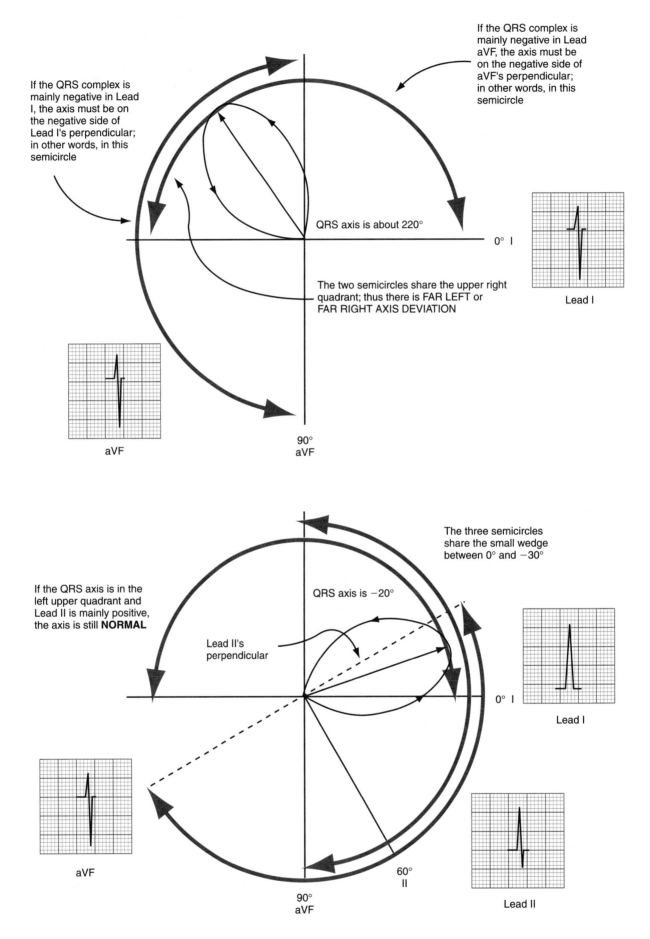

If the QRS complex is mainly negative in Lead I, the axis must be on the negative side of Lead I's perpendicular; in other words, in this semicircle

If the QRS complex is mainly negative in Lead aVF, the axis must be on the negative side of aVF's perpendicular; in other words, in this semicircle

QRS axis is about 220°

The two semicircles share the upper right quadrant; thus there is FAR LEFT or FAR RIGHT AXIS DEVIATION

0° I

Lead I

90° aVF

aVF

If the QRS axis is in the left upper quadrant and Lead II is mainly positive, the axis is still **NORMAL**

The three semicircles share the small wedge between 0° and −30°

QRS axis is −20°

Lead II's perpendicular

0° I

Lead I

60° II

Lead II

90° aVF

aVF

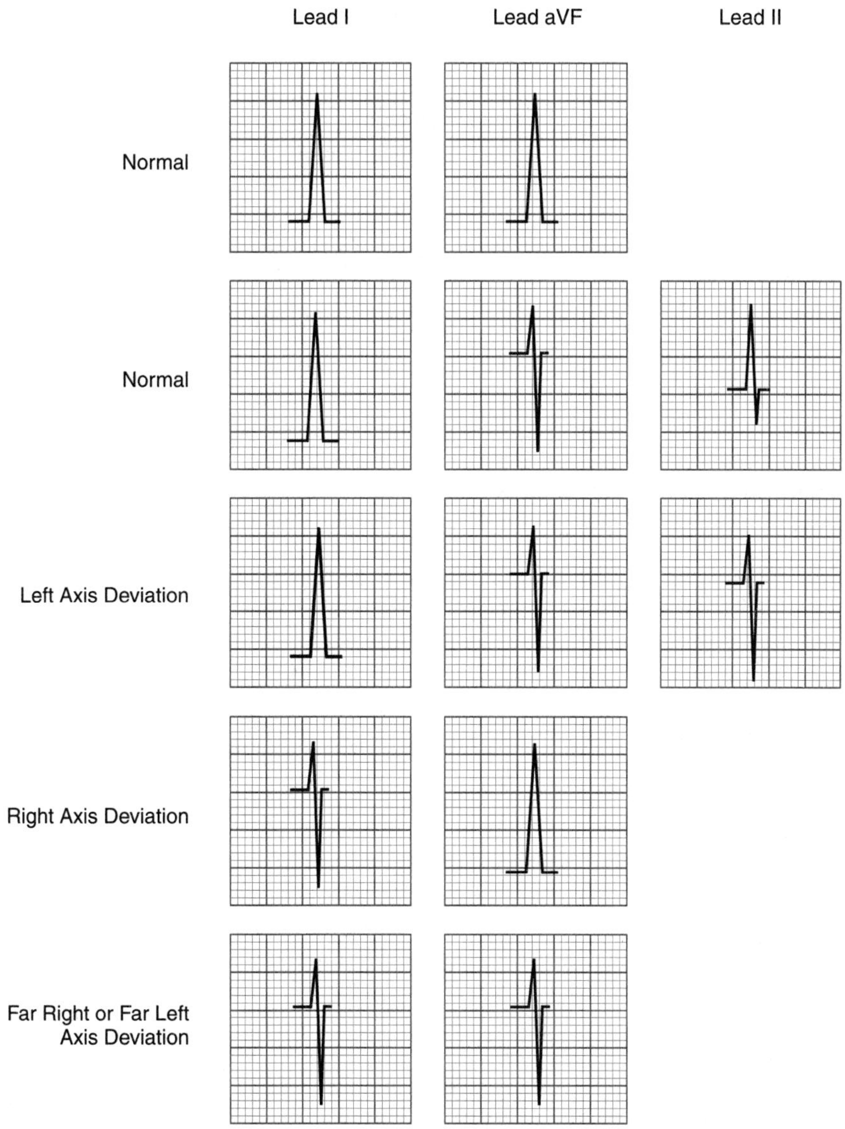

	Lead I	Lead aVF	Lead II

Normal

Normal

Left Axis Deviation

Right Axis Deviation

Far Right or Far Left
Axis Deviation

SUMMARY OF QRS AXES

C.   The chest leads are placed similarly to form a vector loop in the horizontal plane.

D.   The vector loop in the horizontal plane is normally directed anteriorly and leftward, due to the position of the left ventricle.

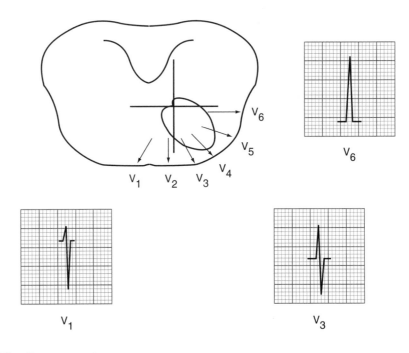

E.   The P wave axis
1.   The normal P wave axis is quite restricted in its range (15°–75°) because of the location of the SA node in the upper right corner of the right atrium.
2.   The P wave should obviously be upright in Leads I and aVF.

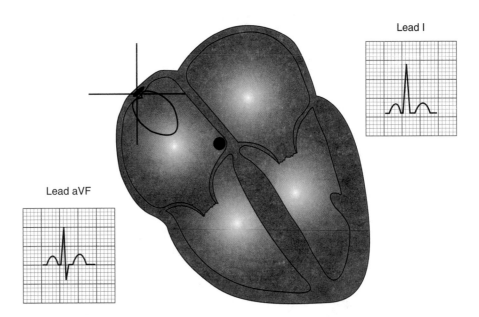

V.   Determining heart rate

A.   If the rhythm is regular, the heart rate can be determined by the distance between complexes.

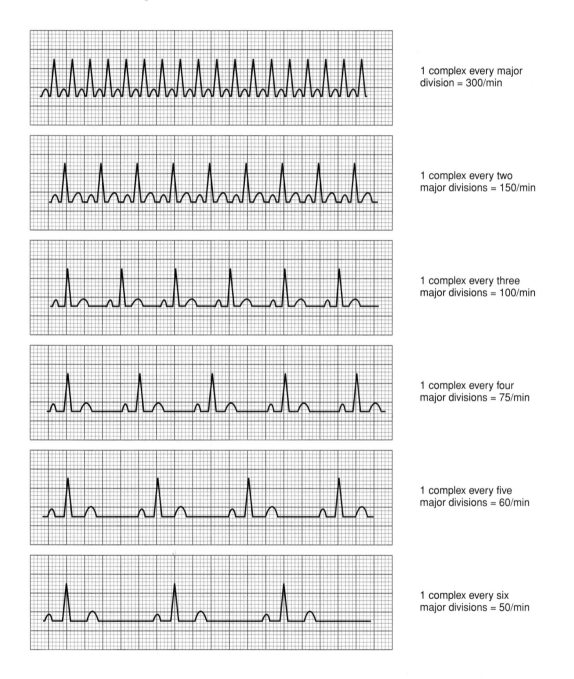

1 complex every major division = 300/min

1 complex every two major divisions = 150/min

1 complex every three major divisions = 100/min

1 complex every four major divisions = 75/min

1 complex every five major divisions = 60/min

1 complex every six major divisions = 50/min

B. If the rhythm is irregular, the rate can be determined by counting the number of beats in 6 seconds and multiplying by 10.

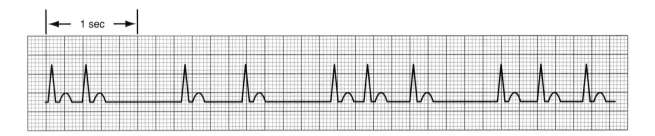

VI. Sinus rhythm

A. Sinus rhythm is defined as:
   1. Regularly recurring P waves of the same morphology
   2. A normal P wave axis
   3. A rate between 60 and 100 beats per minute

B. In addition, if each P wave is followed by a QRS complex, then there is normal sinus rhythm.

Lead I

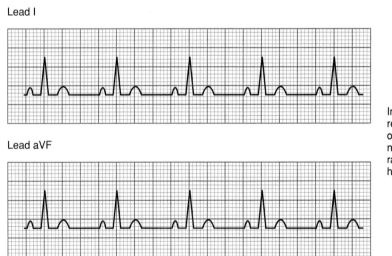

Lead aVF

In this example, there are regularly recurring P waves of similar morphology, a normal P wave axis, and a rate between 60 and 100; hence this is sinus rhythm

VII. Systematic approach to ECG interpretation—a systematic approach is essential: it facilitates the interpretation of complex tracings and assures that no diagnosis is neglected.

    A. Rate
        1. Supraventricular
        2. Ventricular

    B. Rhythm
        1. Supraventricular
        2. Ventricular

    C. Axis
        1. P wave
        2. QRS complex
        3. T wave

    D. P wave morphology

    E. PR interval

    F. QRS complex
        1. Axis
        2. Voltage
        3. Duration
        4. Morphology

    G. ST segment

    H. T wave

    I. QT interval

    J. U wave

VIII. Normal values

Normal Values of ECG Components

	AXIS	INTERVAL
P wave	15° to 75°	—
PR Interval	—	120–200 msec
QRS Complex	−30° to +90°	80–105 msec
T wave	30° to +90°	—
QT interval	—	<1/2 of R–R interval

Day 1 ECG 1

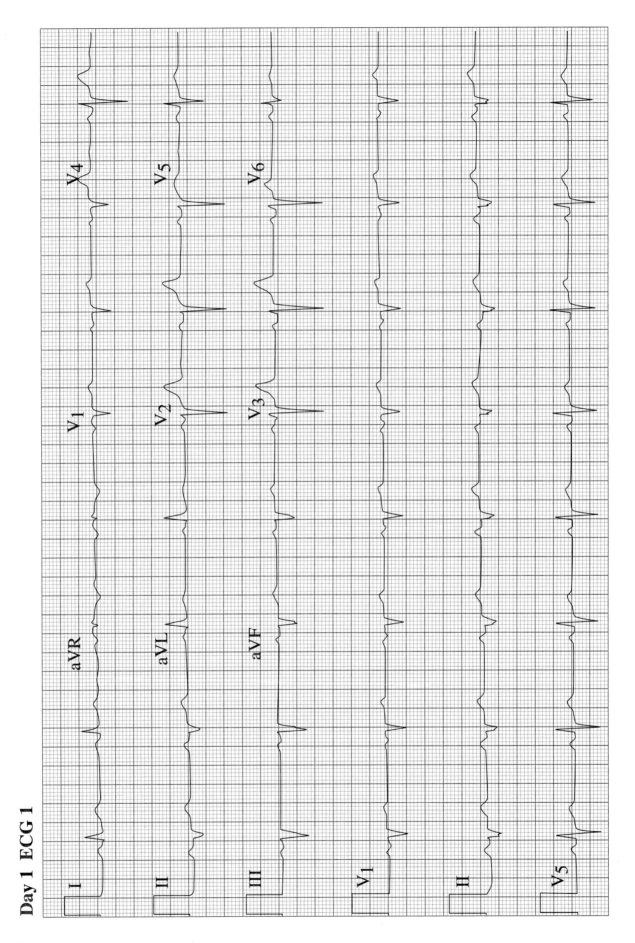

Day 1 ECG 2

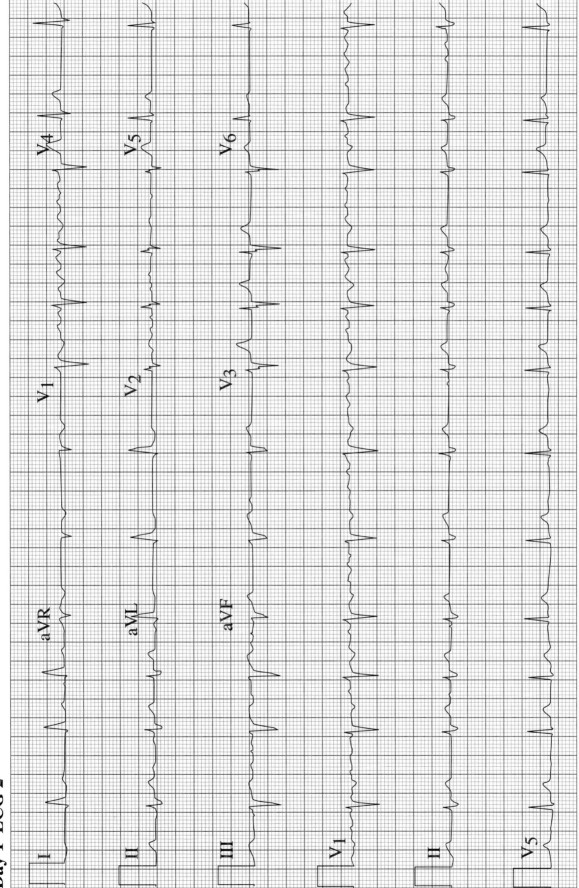

17

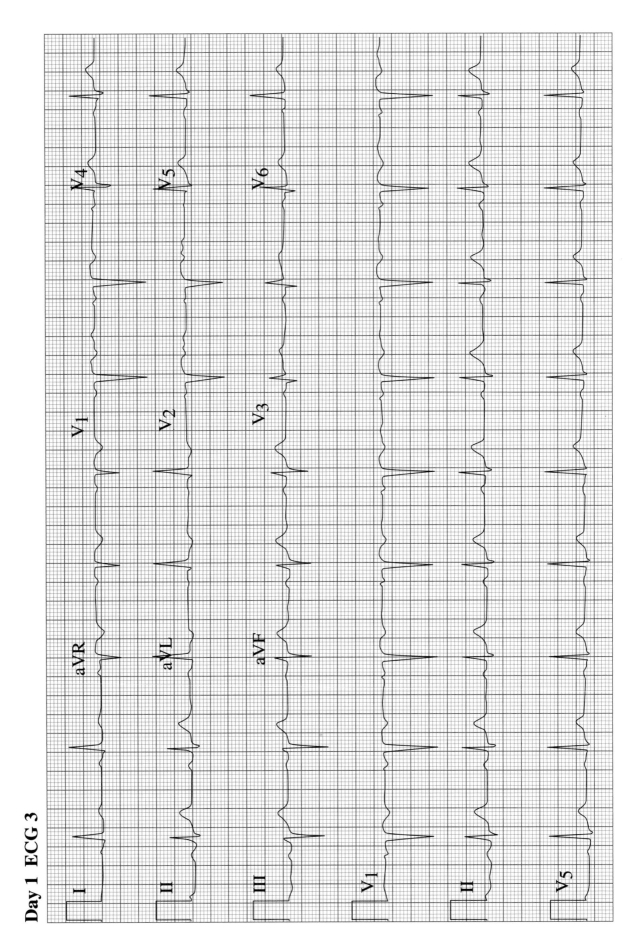

I

II

III

V₁

II

V₅

aVR

aVL

aVF

V₁

V₂

V₃

V₄

V₅

V₆

Day 1 ECG 4

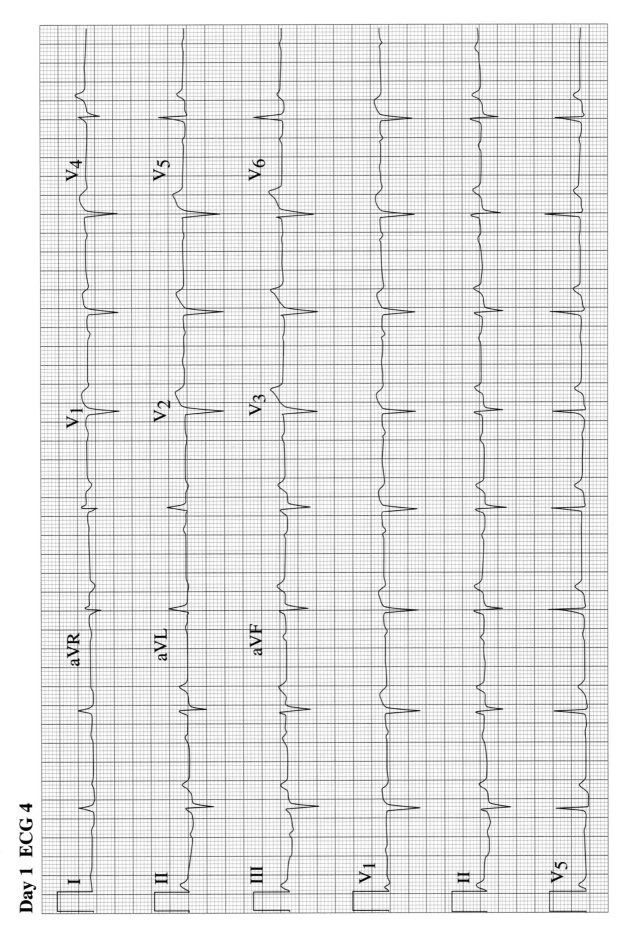

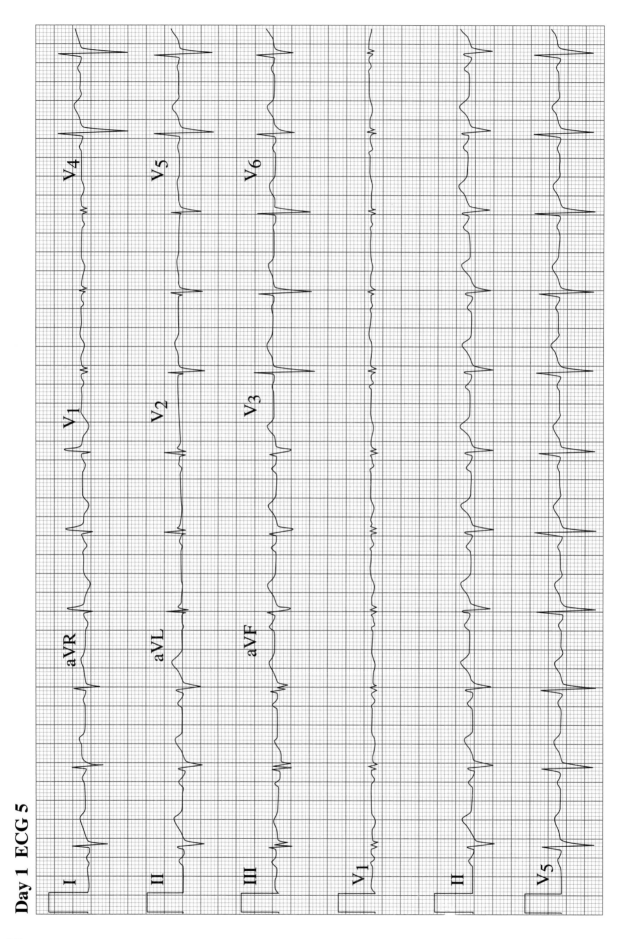

Day 1 ECG 6

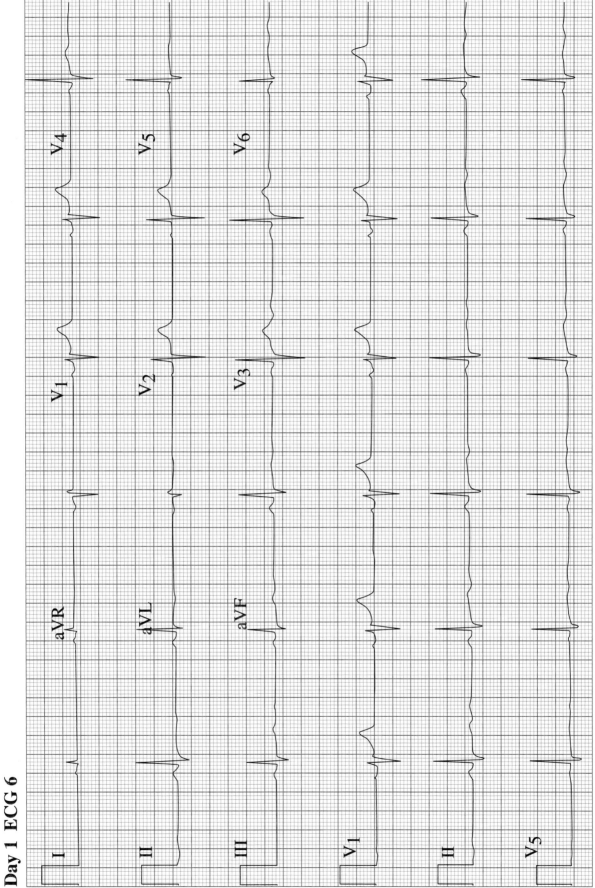

Day 1 ECG 7

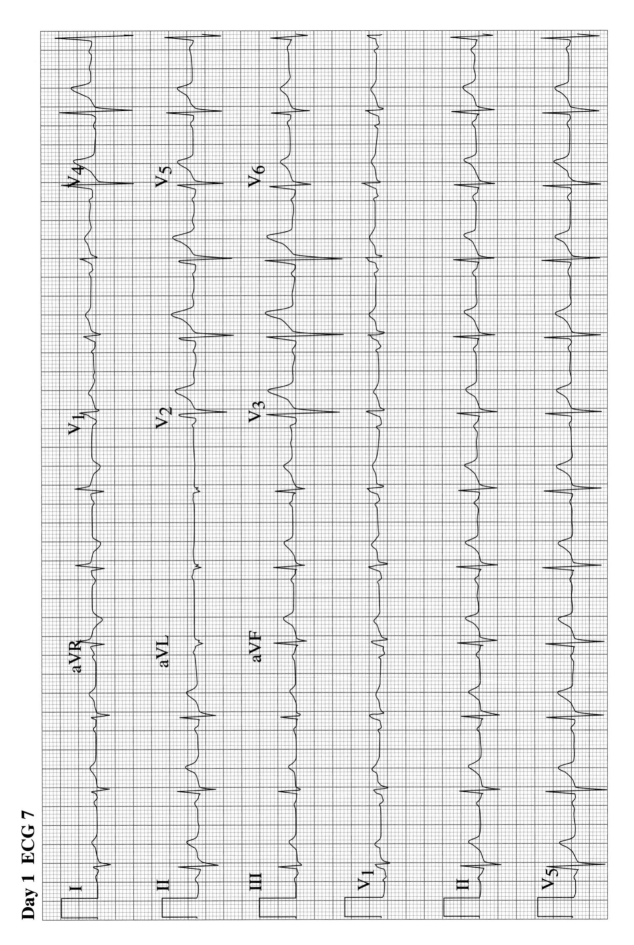

Day 1 ECG 8

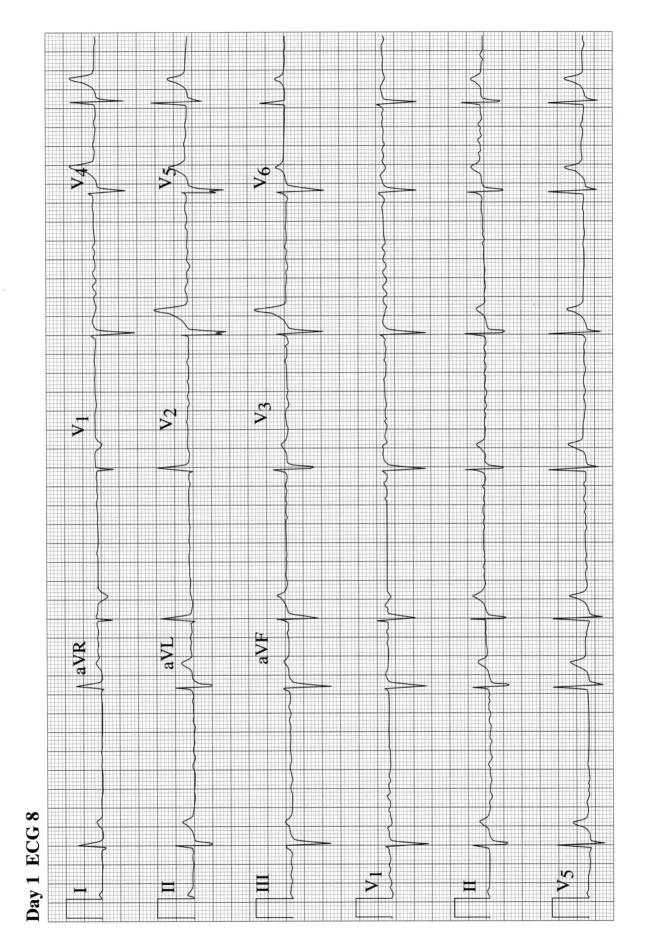

23

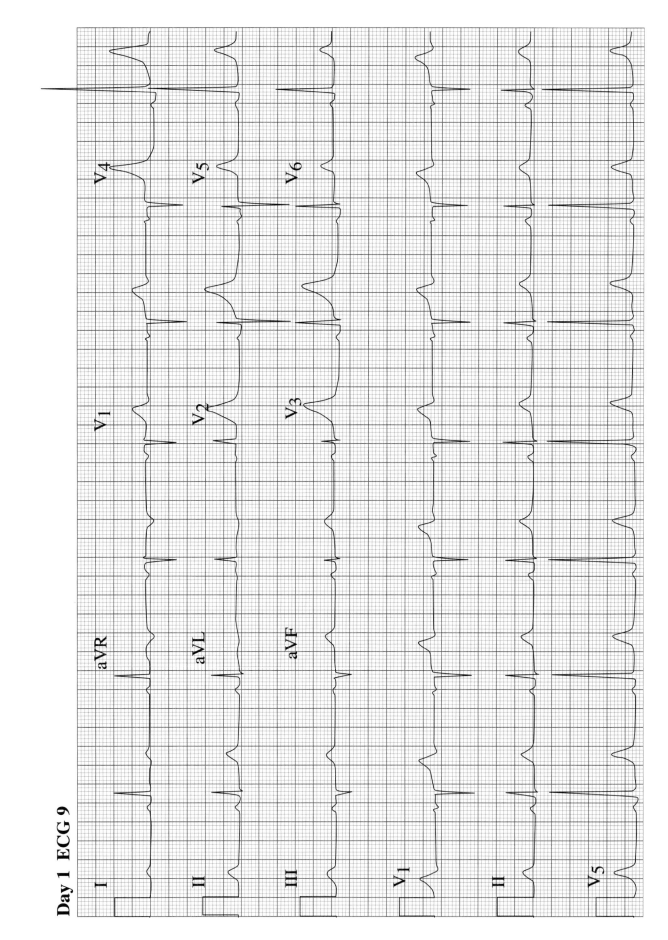

Day 1 ECG 9

24

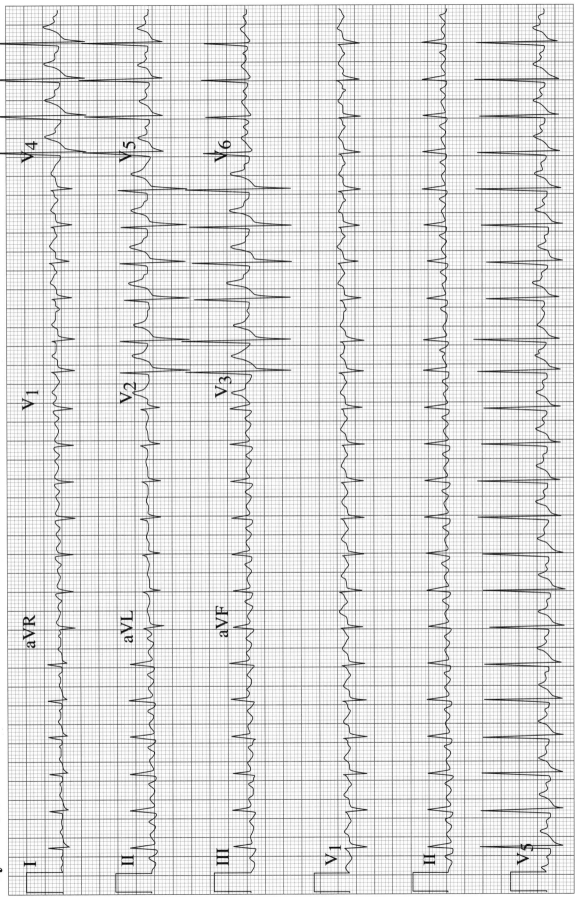

Day 1
ECG Interpretations and Discussion

Day 1 ECG 1
Sinus bradycardia
Left axis deviation
Delayed precordial transition

The QRS complexes are more than 5 major divisions apart, indicating a rate less than 60.

Day 1 ECG 2
Atrial fibrillation
QRS axis = $-30°$

There is an irregular rhythm with an irregular baseline, indicating atrial fibrillation. The heart rate must be determined by averaging the number of beats over a suitable interval, such as 6 or 10 seconds. The QRS complex is upright in I, downward in aVF, and isoelectric in II, indicating a QRS axis of about $-30°$.

Day 1 ECG 3
Sinus rhythm
Anteroseptal MI, age undetermined
Nonspecific ST and T wave changes

The QRS complex is upright in I, downward in aVF, and upright in II, indicating a QRS axis between $0°$ and $-30°$. There are prominent Q waves in V_1–V_4 indicating an old anteroseptal MI. There is mild sagging of the ST segments in several leads and T wave inversion in aVL.

Day 1 ECG 4
Sinus bradycardia
First degree AV block
Left axis deviation
Probable anteroseptal MI, age undetermined
Nonspecific ST and T wave changes

The QRS complexes are more than 5 major divisions apart, indicating a rate less than 60 beats/min. The PR interval is greater than 200 msec. The QRS complex is upright in I, downward in aVF, and downward in II, indicating left axis deviation. There are Q waves in V_1 and V_2, indicating a probable old anteroseptal MI. There is sagging of the ST segments in several leads and T wave inversion in aVL.

Day 1 ECG 5
Normal sinus rhythm
Right superior axis deviation
Delayed precordial transition

The QRS complex is downward in I and aVF, indicating a QRS axis in the right upper quadrant. In the precordial leads, the R wave should be more prominent than the S wave by V_4.

Day 1 ECG 6
Sinus bradycardia

The QRS complexes are more than 5 major divisions apart, indicating a rate less than 60 beats/min.

Day 1 ECG 7
Normal sinus rhythm
Right axis deviation
Probable RVH

The QRS complex is downward in I and upright in aVF, indicating right axis deviation. There are prominent S waves across the precordial leads. This, in the presence of right axis deviation, suggests right ventricular hypertrophy.

Day 1 ECG 8
Atrial fibrillation with slow ventricular response
Left axis deviation

There is an irregular rhythm with an irregular baseline, indicating atrial fibrillation. The average heart rate is less than 60. The QRS complex is upright in I, and downward in aVF and II, indicating left axis deviation.

Day 1 ECG 9
Sinus bradycardia
Nonspecific ST and T wave changes

The QRS complexes are more than 5 major divisions apart, indicating a rate less than 60. There is a small amount of ST segment elevation in several precordial leads, probably indicating early repolarization. It is also possible that the ST changes are from left ventricular hypertrophy, which is suggested by the prominent QRS voltage in V_4 and V_5.

Day 1 ECG 10
Sinus tachycardia

The QRS complexes are almost exactly 2 major divisions apart, indicating a rate of 150.

Day 2

Chamber Abnormalities

I.   General statements

   A.   Echocardiography has become the gold standard for assessing chamber size and wall thickness.

   B.   In general, the sensitivity of the following criteria is moderate (in the range of 50%), and the specificity is very high (> 90%).

II.   Right atrial abnormality

   A.   The amplitude of the P wave must be > 2.5 mm in II, III, or aVF and the morphology must be peaked.

   B.   The P wave axis is frequently > 70°.

Lead I

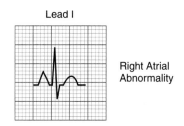

Right Atrial
Abnormality

III.   Left atrial abnormality

   A.   In most forms of acquired LA abnormality, the commonest manifestation is a wide (> 40 msec) and deep (> 1 mm) terminal portion of the P wave in V_1.

   B.   An appearance typical in mitral valvular disease is a "double-humped" P wave, at least 130 msec in duration, in II, III, or aVF.

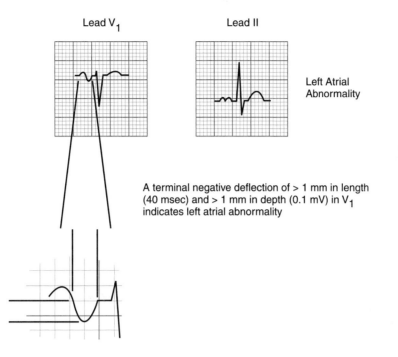

A terminal negative deflection of > 1 mm in length (40 msec) and > 1 mm in depth (0.1 mV) in V_1 indicates left atrial abnormality

IV.   Biatrial abnormality—suggested by a combination of tall P waves in II, III, or aVF, and the terminal negativity in V_1.

V.   Right ventricular hypertrophy (RVH)

   A.   RVH is *suggested* by one or more of the following:
      1.   Right axis deviation
      2.   A tall R wave in V_1 ($\geq$ 7 mm)
      3.   R wave in V_1 + S wave in V_6 $\geq$ 10 mm
      4.   R/S ratio in V_1 $\geq$ 1
      5.   Incomplete RBBB pattern
      6.   Right atrial abnormality
      7.   S > R in V_6

   B.   The diagnosis of RVH requires exclusion of the other causes of a tall R wave in V_1 (see Day 9).

   C.   RVH in patients with acquired pulmonary disease tends to present in a different form:
      1.   Deep S waves are present across the precordium.
      2.   The R wave transition across the precordium is delayed.
      3.   Right axis deviation and right atrial abnormality are frequently present.
      4.   Low voltage may be present.

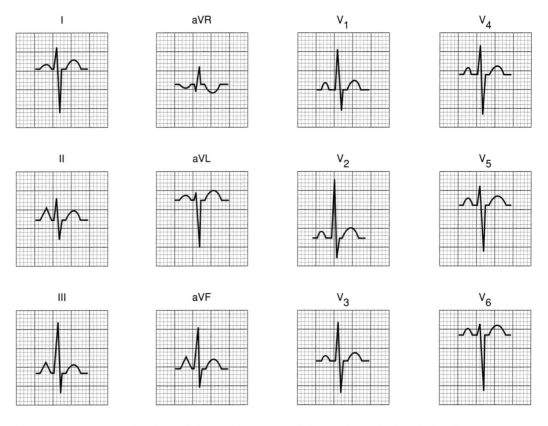

Right ventricular hypertrophy with a tall R wave in V_1, right atrial abnormality, and right axis deviation

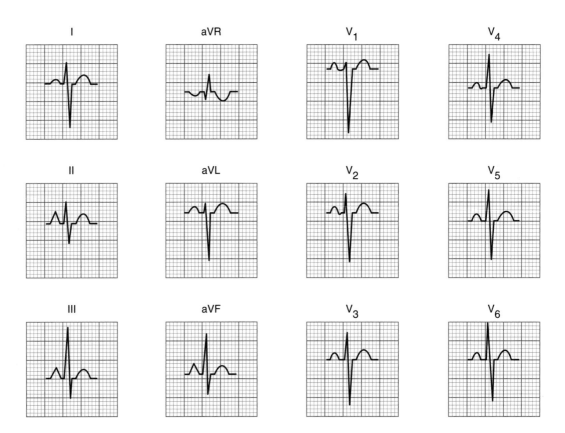

Right ventricular hypertrophy with deep S waves across the precordium, right atrial abnormality, and right axis deviation consistent with pulmonary disease

VI. Left ventricular hypertrophy (LVH)—any of the following are consistent with LVH.

    A. Precordial leads (any of the following)
       1. S wave in V_1 + R wave in V_5 or V_6 > 35 mm in adults (> 30 years)
       2. R wave in V_5 or V_6 > 26 mm

    B. Limb leads (any of the following)
       1. R wave in I > 14 mm
       2. R wave in aVL > 11 mm

    C. LVH is frequently accompanied by ST segment and T wave abnormalities, sometimes referred to as a "strain" pattern, but more appropriately as repolarization abnormalities.

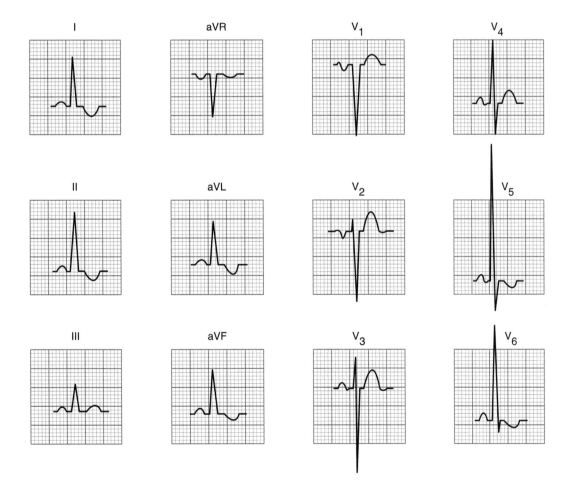

LVH with repolarization abnormalities. Note the large voltage in multiple leads and the diffuse ST and T wave abnormalities. There is also left atrial abnormality in V_1.

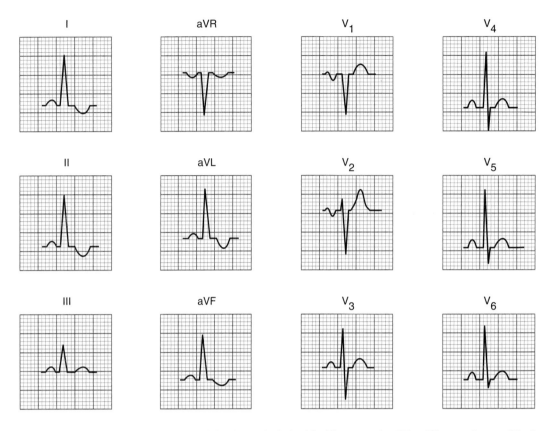

LVH with increased voltage only in the limb leads, particularly aVL. There are also ST and T wave abnormalities in the limb leads and left atrial abnormality in V_1.

VII. Low voltage

    A. Definition
        1. No QRS complex with an absolute value $\geq$ 0.1 mv (10 mm)
        2. Or, no limb lead QRS $\geq$ 0.05 mv (5 mm) (so-called low voltage in the limb leads)

    B. Causes
        1. Decreased voltage production by the myocardium
            a. Restrictive cardiomyopathies (amyloidosis, sarcoidosis, etc.)
            b. Hypothyroidism
        2. Increased impedance between the voltage-producing source (the myocardium) and the ECG leads
            a. Fat (obesity)
            b. Air (COPD, tension pneumothorax)
            c. Water (pericardial or pleural effusion, ascites)

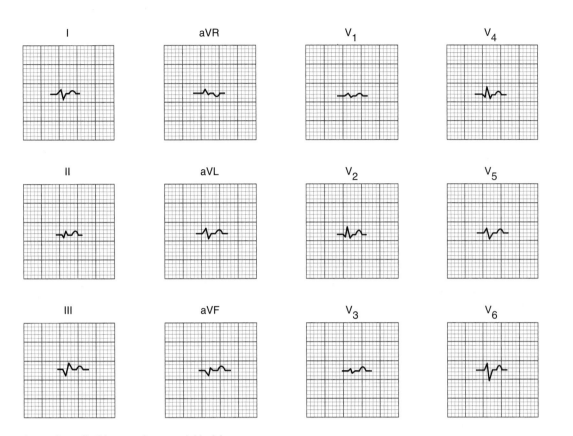

Low voltage (in this case, from amyloidosis)

Day 2 ECG 1

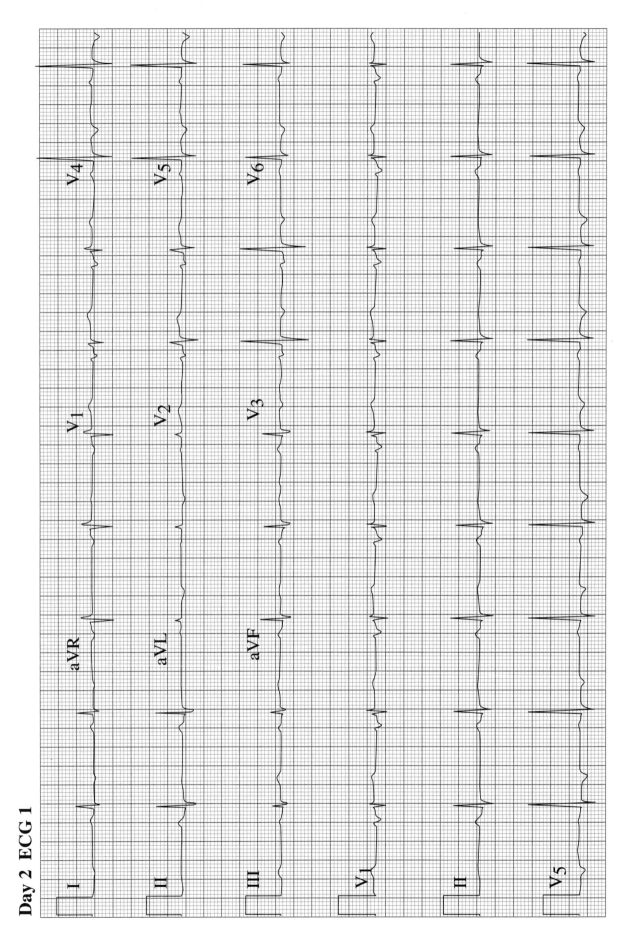

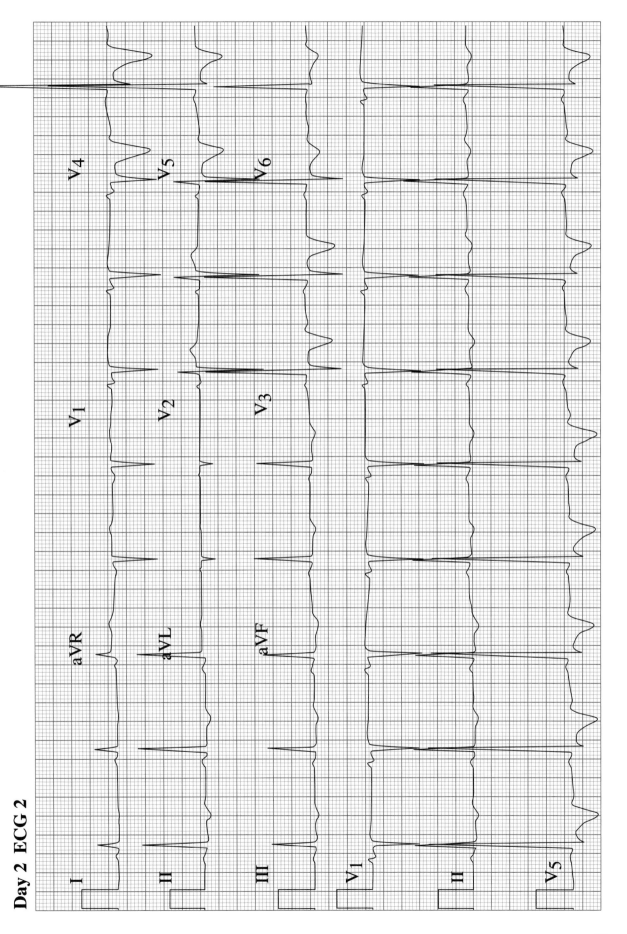

Day 2 ECG 2

I aVR V1 V4

II aVL V2 V5

III aVF V3 V6

V1

II

V5

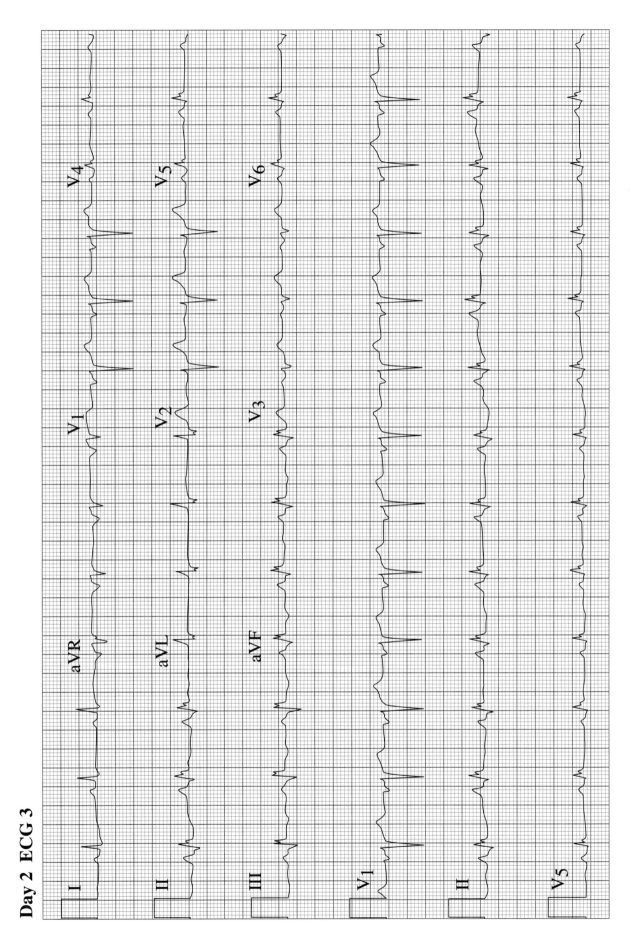

Day 2 ECG 3

36

Day 2 ECG 4

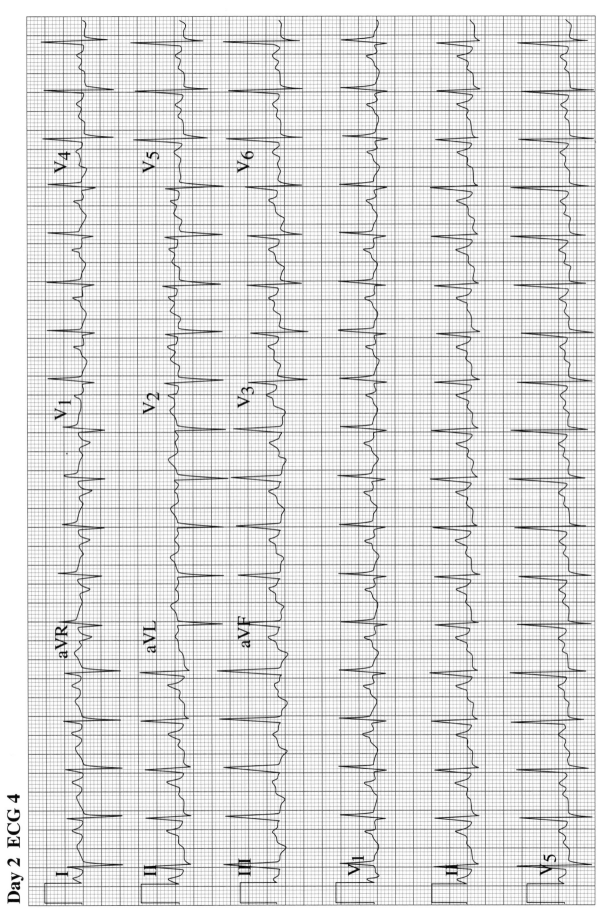

Day 2 ECG 5

** Chest leads at half standard **

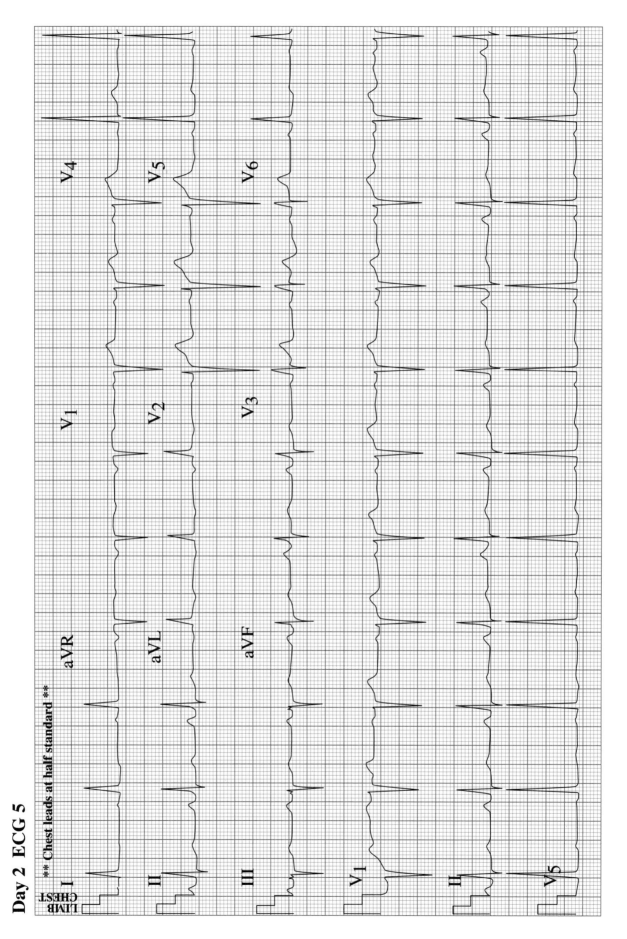

Day 2 ECG 6

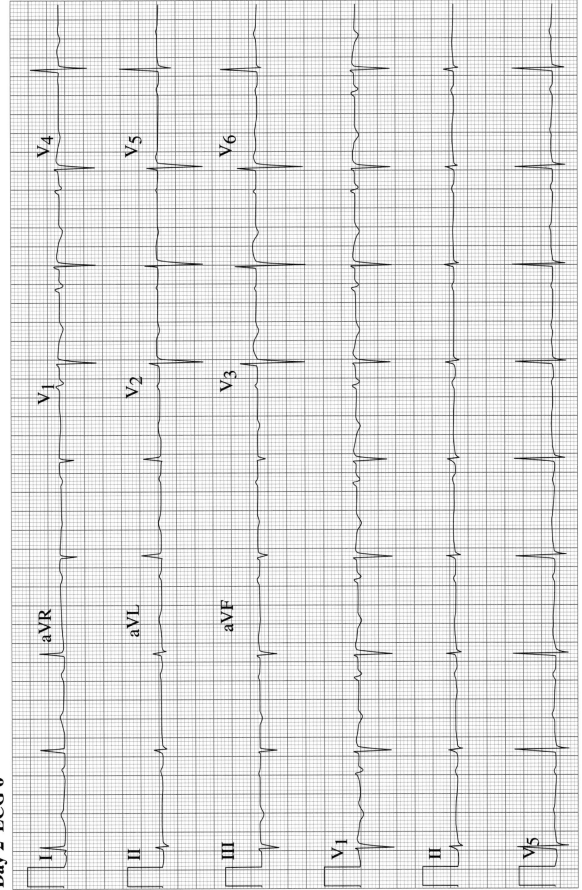

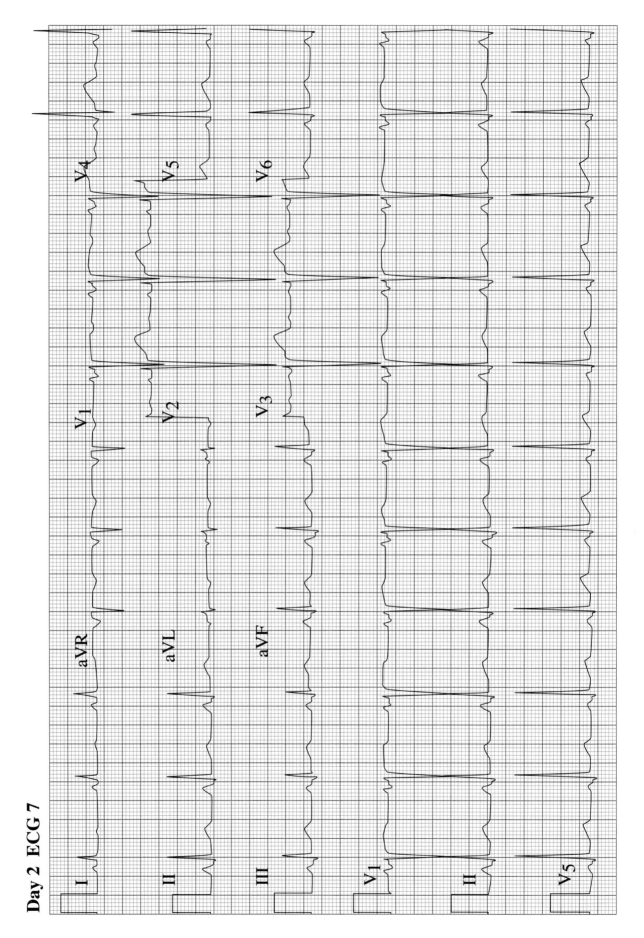

Day 2 ECG 8

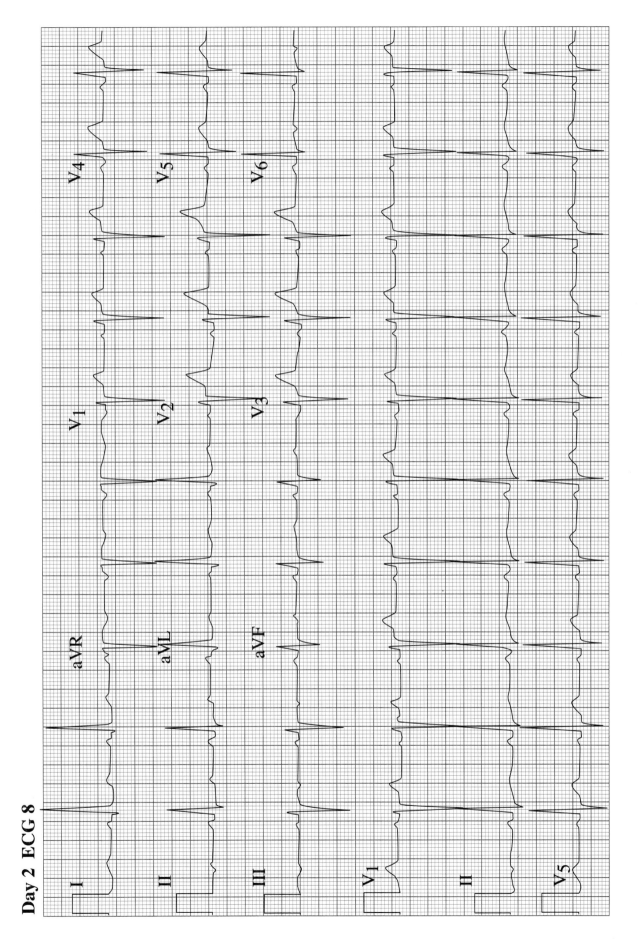

Day 2 ECG 9

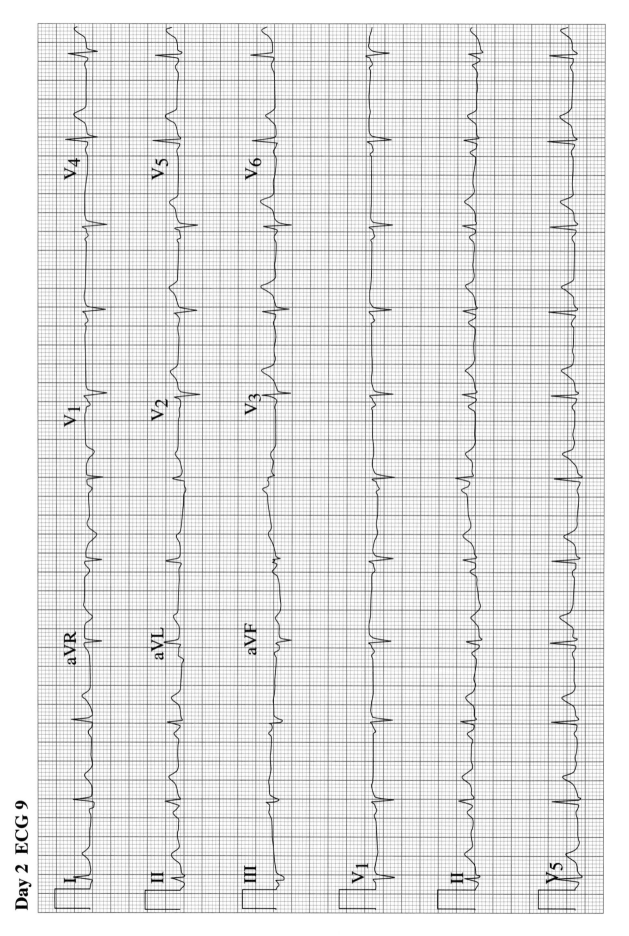

Day 2 ECG 10

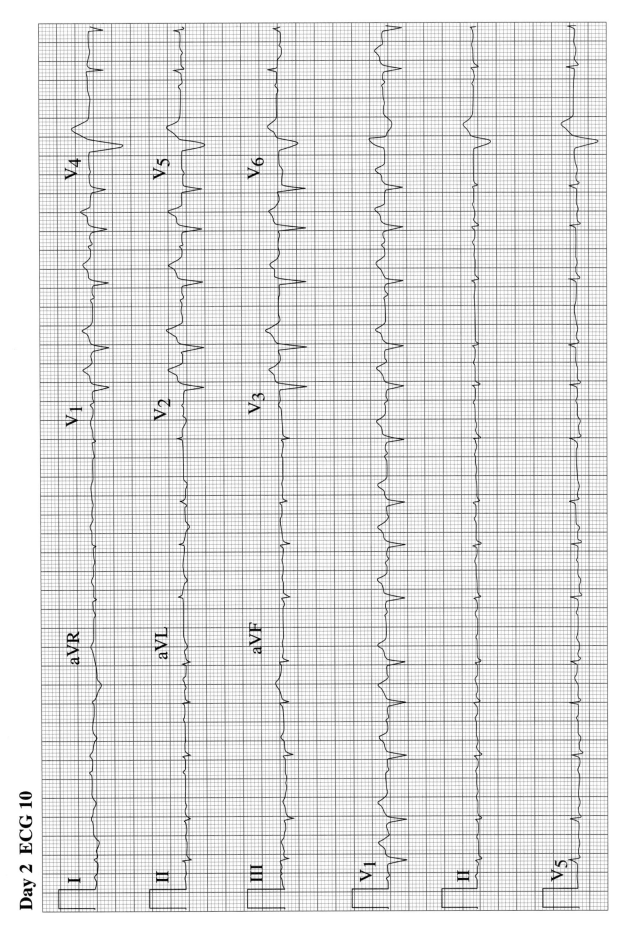

Day 2
ECG Interpretations and Discussion

Day 2 ECG 1
   Normal sinus rhythm
   Left atrial abnormality
   Nonspecific T wave changes

The terminal portion of the P wave is inverted and at least 1 mm deep and wide in V_1. There is widespread T wave inversion.

Day 2 ECG 2
   Normal sinus rhythm
   Left ventricular hypertrophy with repolarization abnormalities

There are voltage criteria for left ventricular hypertrophy in the precordial leads, and widespread ST depression and T wave inversion.

Day 2 ECG 3
   Normal sinus rhythm
   Biatrial abnormality
   Inferolateral MI, age undetermined

The P waves are tall and pointed in II and aVF, and there is significant terminal negativity in V_1, indicating biatrial abnormality. There are significant Q waves in the inferior leads, small Q waves in V_5 and V_6, and loss of R wave height in V_3–V_6, indicating an inferolateral MI.

Day 2 ECG 4
   Sinus tachycardia
   Right axis deviation
   Right atrial abnormality
   Probable RVH with repolarization abnormalities

The interval between the QRS complexes is less than three major divisions, indicating sinus tachycardia. The QRS complex is downward in I and upright in aVF, indicating right axis deviation. The P waves are tall and pointed in II and aVF, indicating right atrial abnormality. These findings, along with tall R waves in V_1, strongly suggest right ventricular hypertrophy. The ST segment and T wave changes are associated with the RVH.

Day 2 ECG 5
   Normal sinus rhythm
   Left ventricular hypertrophy with repolarization abnormalities

The chest leads are at half standard, as indicated by the notation in the upper left corner of the tracing and by the "stair step" calibration mark at the beginning of each lead. Therefore, there are voltage criteria for left ventricular hypertrophy in the precordial leads.

Day 2 ECG 6
Sinus bradycardia
Left atrial abnormality
First degree AV block

The interval between the QRS complexes is greater than five major divisions, indicating sinus bradycardia. There is a prominent terminal negative deflection of the P wave in V_1, indicating left atrial abnormality. The PR interval is greater than 200 msec.

Day 2 ECG 7
Normal sinus rhythm
Right atrial abnormality
LVH with repolarization abnormalities

The P waves are tall and pointed in II and aVF, indicating right atrial abnormality. There are voltage criteria for left ventricular hypertrophy in the precordial leads.

Day 2 ECG 8
Normal sinus rhythm
LVH with repolarization abnormalities

There are voltage criteria for left ventricular hypertrophy in the limb leads.

Day 2 ECG 9
Normal sinus rhythm
Low voltage

No QRS complex has an absolute value of more than 10 mm, indicating low voltage. The clinical cause of the low voltage is not clear from this tracing.

Day 2 ECG 10
Sinus tachycardia with frequent atrial extrasystoles and occasional ventricular
    extrasystoles
Low voltage
Probable anteroseptal MI, age undetermined

There are frequent early narrow QRS complexes consistent with atrial extrasystoles. There is one wide QRS complex consistent with a ventricular extrasystole. No QRS complex has an absolute value of more than 10 mm, indicating low voltage. There are prominent Q waves in V_1–V_4, suggesting an anterior MI. However, this patient had an endomyocardial biopsy which demonstrated cardiac amyloidosis. This condition is responsible for the low voltage and the "pseudoinfarction" pattern. At a subsequent autopsy, the coronary arteries were normal.

Day 3

Intraventricular Conduction Defects

I. Right bundle branch block (RBBB)

    A. QRS $\geq$ 120 msec

    B. RSR′ in V_1, V_2, or V_{3R} (initial R wave is missing in concomitant antero-septal MI)

    C. Delayed intrinsicoid deflection time (IDT) (see page 48) in V_1, V_2, or V_{3R}

    D. Wide S wave in I and V_6

II. Left bundle branch block (LBBB)

    A. QRS $\geq$ 120 msec

    B. Delayed IDT in I and V_6

    C. Broad monophasic R wave in I and V_6

III. Nonspecific intraventricular conduction defect (IVCD)

    A. QRS $\geq$ 120 msec

    B. QRS pattern fits neither RBBB or LBBB

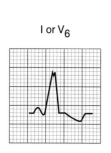

I or V$_6$

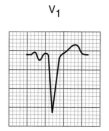

V$_1$

Delayed IDT in I or V$_6$

Monophasic R in I or V$_6$

V$_1$

I or V$_6$

QRS ≥ 120
Neither LBBB or RBBB

Nonspecific IVCD

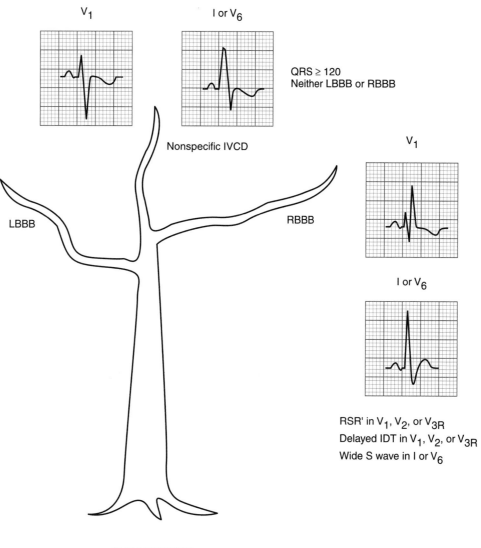

LBBB

RBBB

V$_1$

I or V$_6$

RSR' in V$_1$, V$_2$, or V$_{3R}$
Delayed IDT in V$_1$, V$_2$, or V$_{3R}$
Wide S wave in I or V$_6$

THE IVCD TREE
QRS ≥ 120 msec

The intrinsicoid deflection time is the time from the onset of the QRS to the peak of the major QRS deflection. It should be < 40 msec.

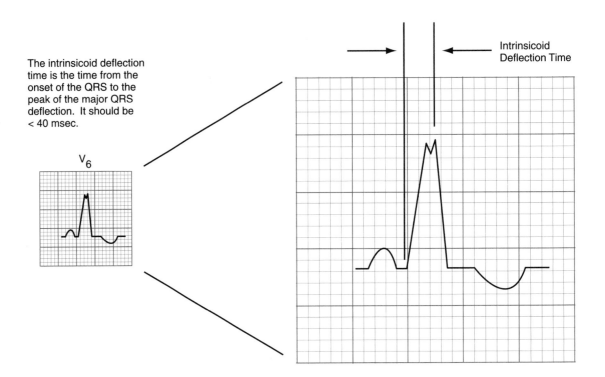

Prolongation of the intrinsicoid deflection time in V$_6$ in LBBB

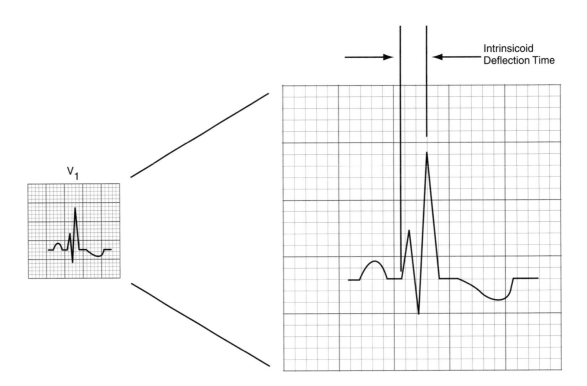

Prolongation of the intrinsicoid deflection time in V$_1$ in RBBB

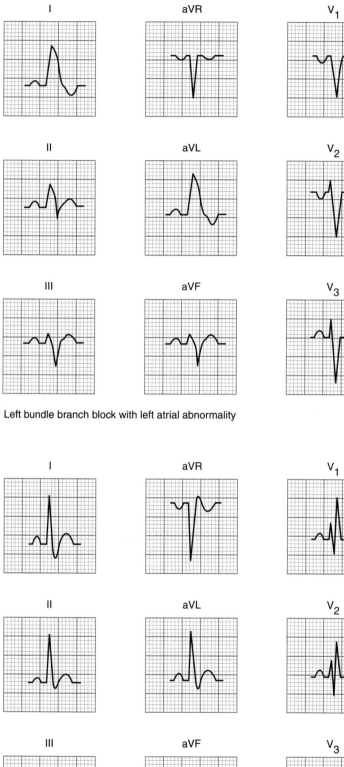
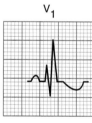
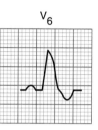
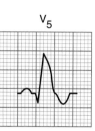

I	aVR	V₁	V₄
II	aVL	V₂	V₅
III	aVF	V₃	V₆

Left bundle branch block with left atrial abnormality

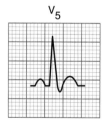
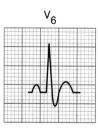
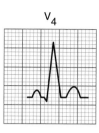

I	aVR	V₁	V₄
II	aVL	V₂	V₅
III	aVF	V₃	V₆

Right bundle branch block

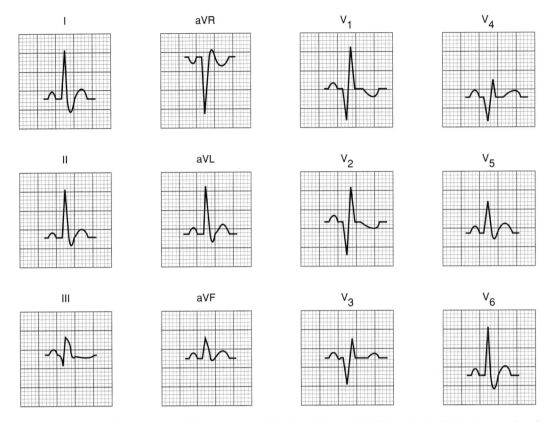

Right bundle branch block with a previous anteroseptal MI. Note that the initial R wave in V_1–V_4 has been replaced by a Q wave.

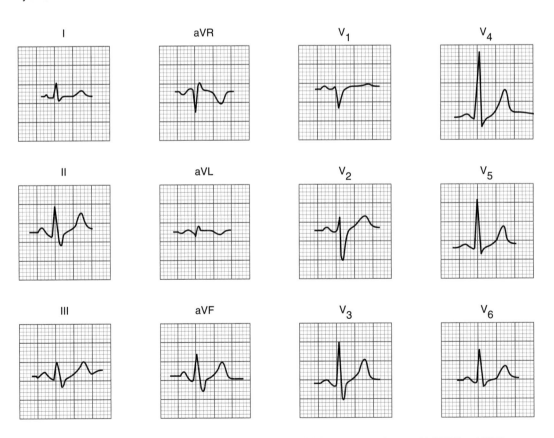

An ECG with QRS complexes > 120 msec, but with features which are not consistent with RBBB or LBBB; therefore this is a nonspecific IVCD

IV. Left anterior fascicular block (LAFB)

    A. Left axis deviation > 45°

    B. Tiny Q waves in I or aVL

    C. Usually slightly prolonged QRS duration (> 90 msec)

    D. No other causes for LAD (e.g., LVH, inferior MI, chronic lung disease)

V. Left posterior fascicular block (LPFB)

    A. Right axis deviation > 100°

    B. Deep S wave in I and a small Q wave in III

    C. Usually slightly prolonged QRS duration (> 90 msec)

    D. No other causes for RAD (e.g., RVH, chronic lung disease, lateral MI)

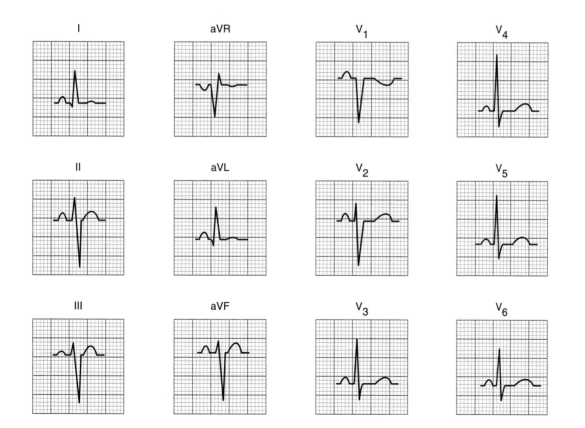

Left anterior fascicular block

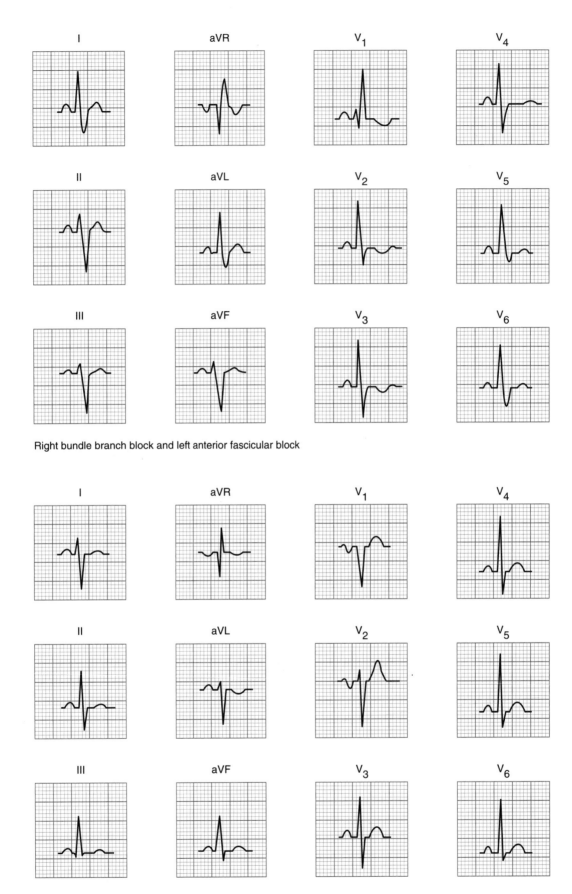

Right bundle branch block and left anterior fascicular block

Left posterior fascicular block

Day 3 ECG 1

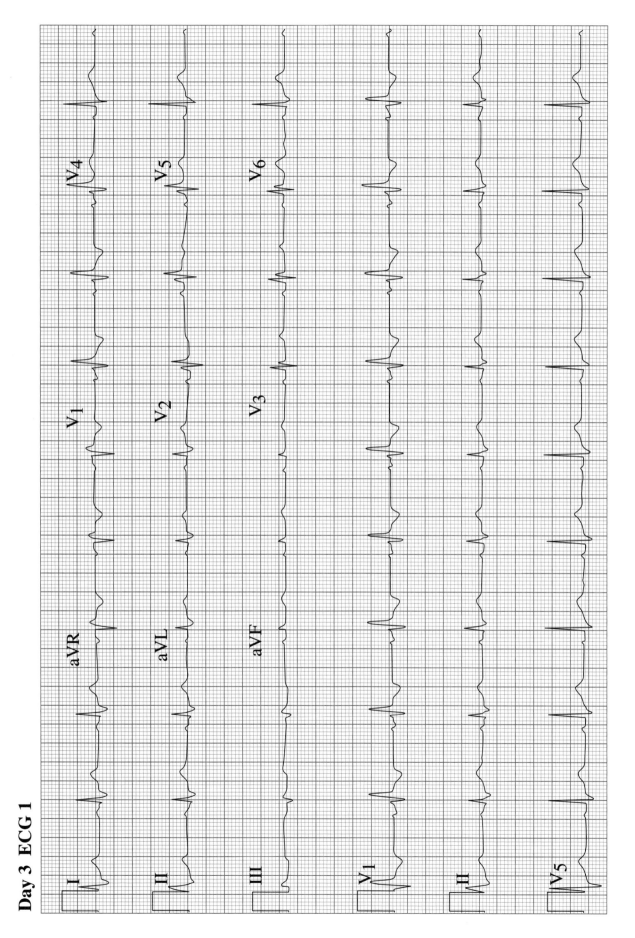

Day 3 ECG 2

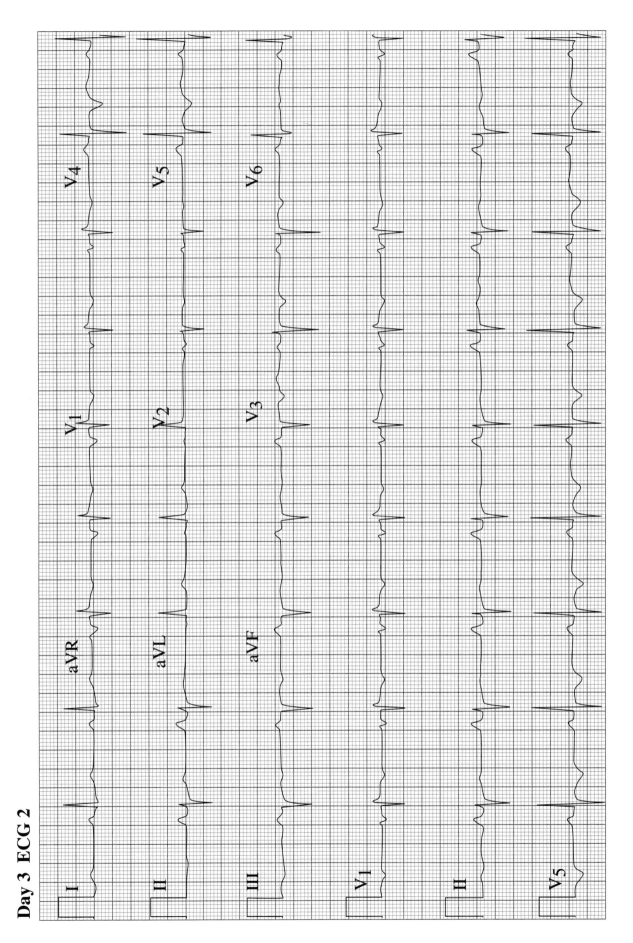

Day 3 ECG 3

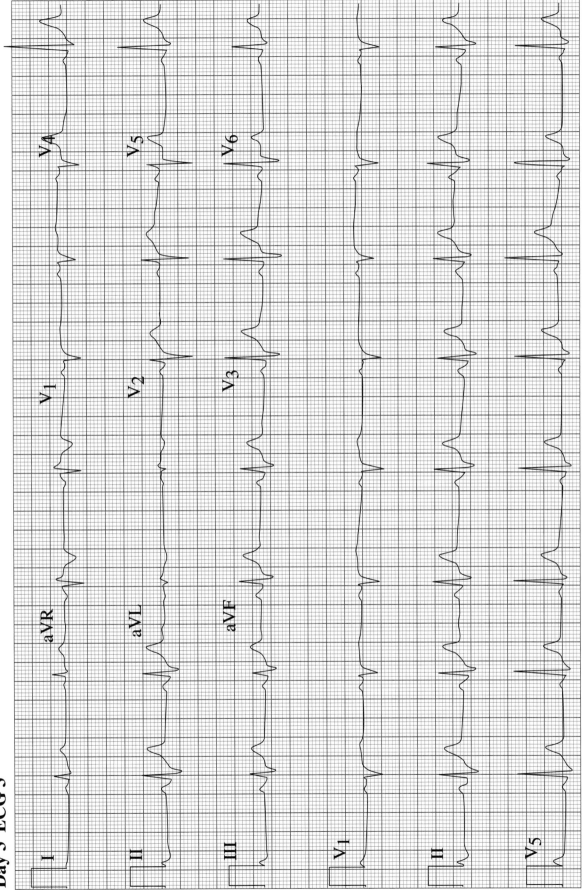

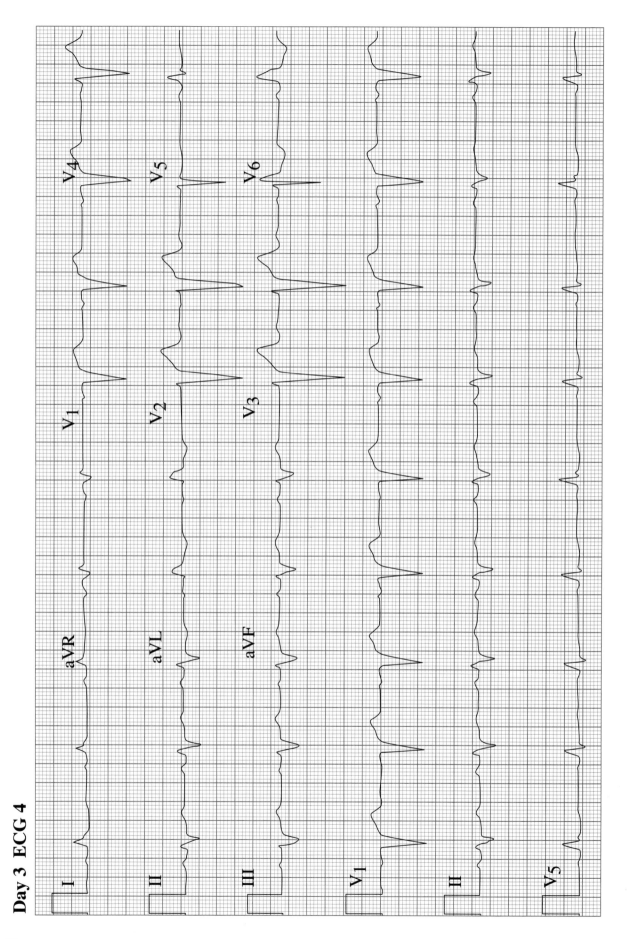

Day 3 ECG 5

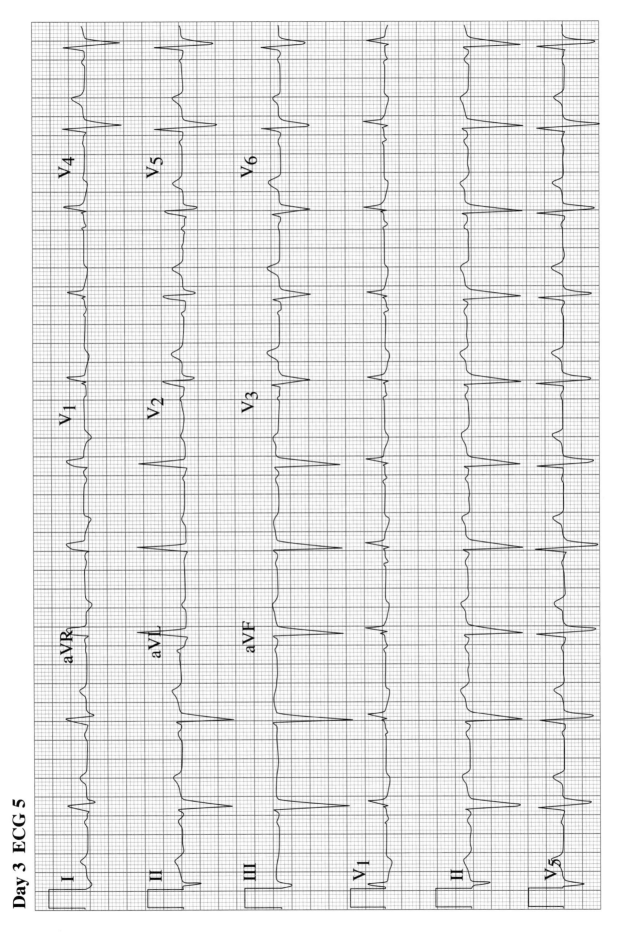

Day 3 ECG 6

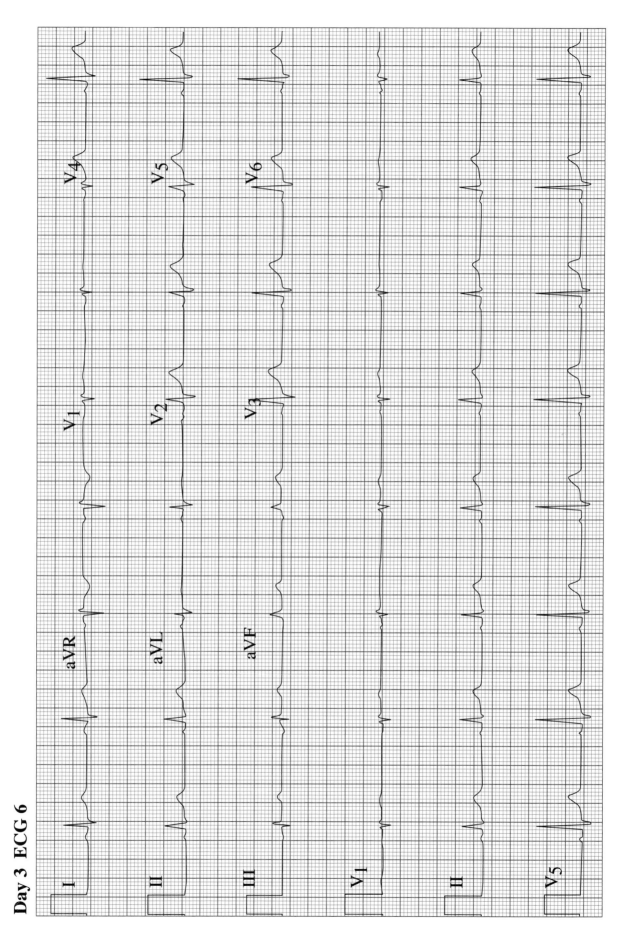

Day 3 ECG 7

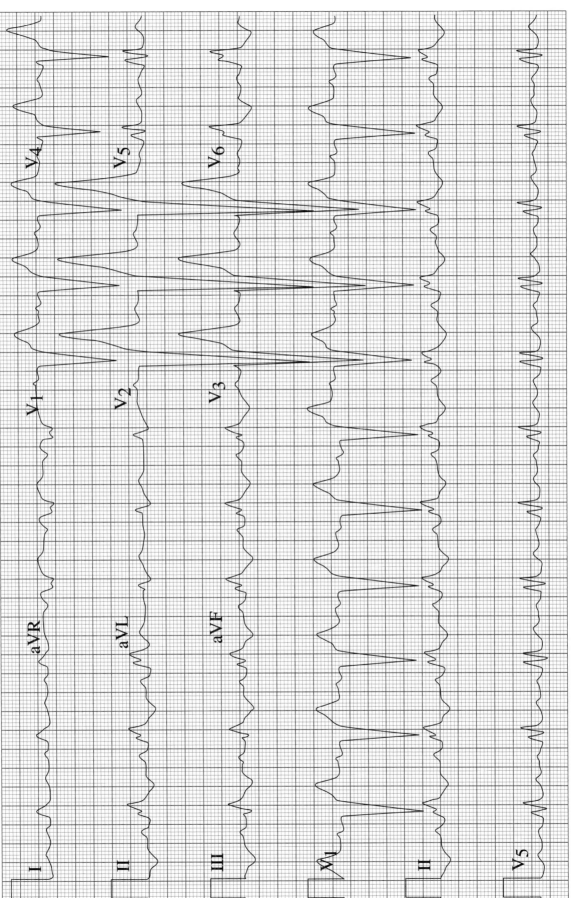

Day 3 ECG 8

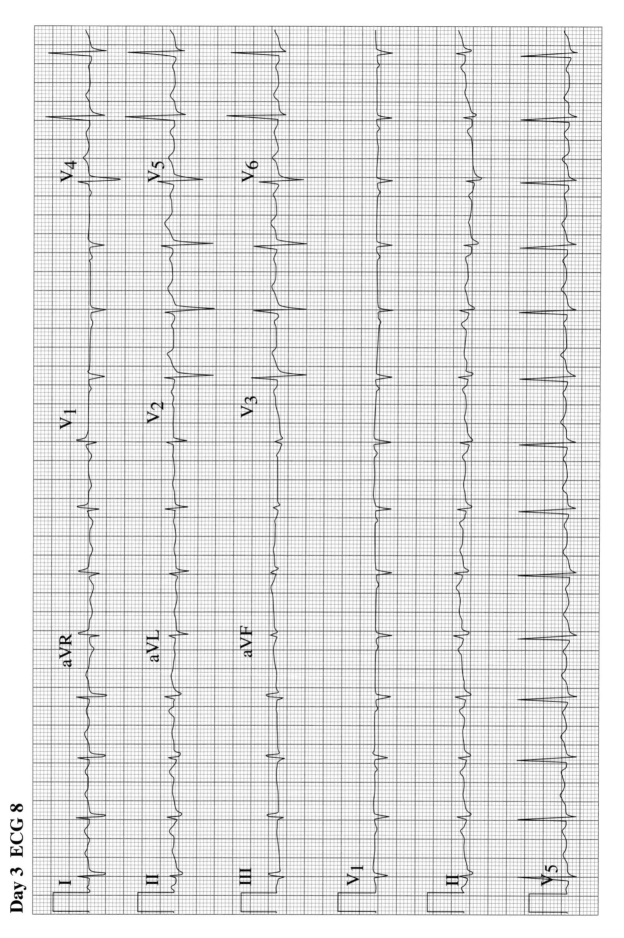

Day 3 ECG 9

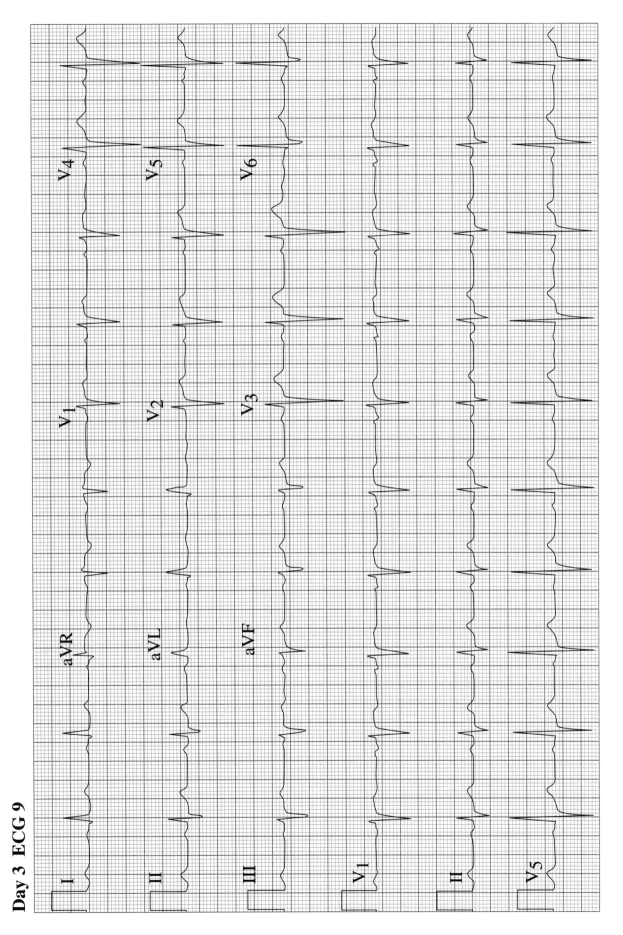

Day 3 ECG10

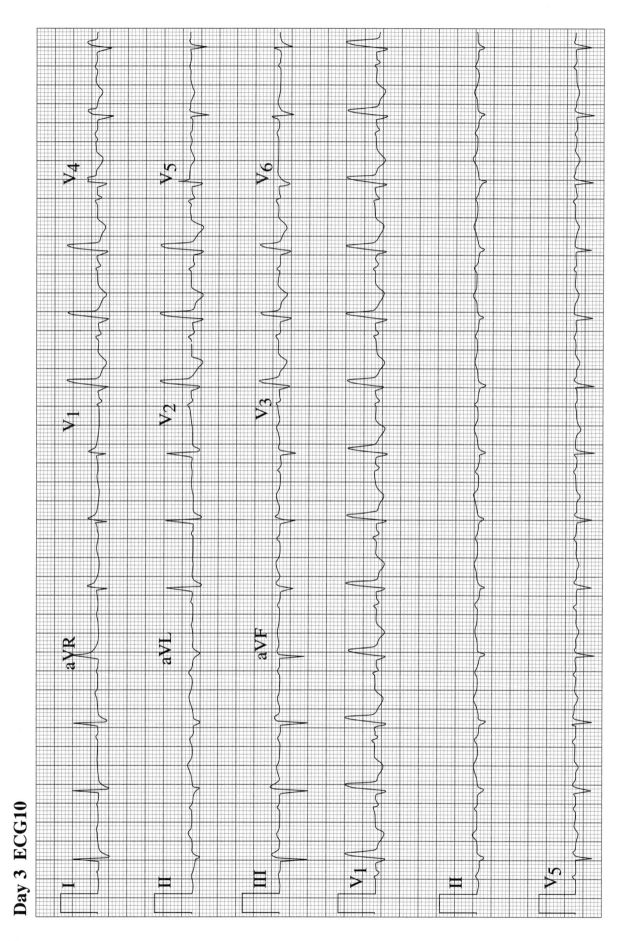

62

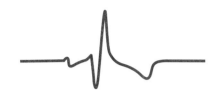

Day 3
ECG Interpretations and Discussion

Day 3 ECG 1
   Normal sinus rhythm
   Right bundle branch block

The QRS complexes are greater than 120 msec, there is a delayed intrinsicoid deflection time in V_1, an RSR′ pattern in V_1, and wide S waves in I and V_6, all consistent with right bundle branch block.

Day 3 ECG 2
   Normal sinus rhythm
   Biatrial abnormality
   Incomplete right bundle branch block
   Nonspecific T wave changes

The P waves are tall and pointed in II and aVF, and there is significant terminal negativity in V_1, indicating biatrial abnormality. The QRS complexes have the morphology of right bundle branch block, but are only slightly prolonged (more than 105 but less than 120 msec). There are diffuse T wave abnormalities.

Day 3 ECG 3
   Sinus bradycardia
   Nonspecific intraventricular conduction defect

The QRS complexes are greater than 120 msec, but criteria for right or left bundle branch block are not present, consistent with a nonspecific intraventricular conduction defect.

Day 3 ECG 4
   Sinus bradycardia
   Left bundle branch block

The QRS complexes are greater than 120 msec, the intrinsicoid deflection time is prolonged in I and V_6, and there is a monophasic R wave in those leads, consistent with left bundle branch block.

Day 3 ECG 5
   Normal sinus rhythm
   Left anterior fascicular block
   Right bundle branch block

The QRS complex is upright in I, downward in aVF, and quite negative in II, indicating significant left axis deviation. There are tiny Q waves in I and aVL. The QRS complexes are greater than 120 msec, there is a delayed intrinsicoid deflection time in V_1, an RSR′ pattern in V_1, and wide S waves in V_6, all consistent with left anterior fascicular block and right bundle branch block.

Day 3 ECG 6
    Sinus bradycardia
    Incomplete right bundle branch block

The QRS complexes have the morphology of right bundle branch block, but are only slightly prolonged (more than 105 but less than 120 msec).

Day 3 ECG 7
    Normal sinus rhythm
    Left bundle branch block

The QRS complexes are greater than 120 msec, the intrinsicoid deflection time is prolonged in I and V_6, and there is a monophasic R wave in those leads, consistent with a left bundle branch block.

Day 3 ECG 8
    Normal sinus rhythm
    Right axis deviation
    Left posterior fascicular block

The QRS complex is downward in I and upright in aVF, indicating right axis deviation. There is a deep S wave in I and a tiny Q wave in III, and there is a slight prolongation of the QRS duration. There are no other factors obviously responsible for right axis deviation. These findings are consistent with left posterior fascicular block.

Day 3 ECG 9
    Normal sinus rhythm
    Nonspecific intraventricular conduction defect

The QRS complexes are greater than 120 msec, but criteria for right or left bundle branch block are not present, consistent with a nonspecific intraventricular conduction defect.

Day 3 ECG 10
    Normal sinus rhythm
    Right bundle branch block
    Anteroseptal MI, age undetermined
    Inferior MI, age undetermined

The QRS complexes are greater than 120 msec, there is a delayed intrinsicoid deflection time in V_1 and wide S waves in I and V_6, consistent with right bundle branch block. The initial R wave in V_1 has been replaced by a Q wave, and there are also Q waves in V_2–V_5, indicating an anterior MI. There are also Q waves in II, III, and aVF, indicating an inferior MI. It is crucial to note that myocardial infarctions can be interpreted in spite of an underlying right bundle branch block.

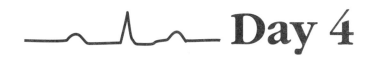 **Day 4**

SA and AV Nodal Conduction Abnormalities

I. Intracardiac electrograms

   A. Conduction disturbances in the surface ECG have their genesis in specific locations in the conduction system.

   B. Surface ECG disturbances are more clearly appreciated by concomitant analysis of the intracardiac electrogram.

   C. Components of the intracardiac electrogram (see page 66)
      1. SA node
         a. There is no surface ECG representation of SA nodal depolarization; a recurrent, normal axis P wave *implies* that the SA node is responsible.
         b. Careful recordings from a tiny area in the upper right portion of the right atrium have demonstrated SA nodal activity preceding atrial depolarization.
      2. Atria
         a. Atrial depolarization produces the P wave on the surface ECG.
         b. The P wave axis is demonstrative of the direction of atrial depolarization.
      3. AV node
         a. The AV node is responsible for most of the delay between the wave and the QRS complex.
         b. On the intracardiac electrogram, the delay in the AV node is represented by the P wave to His bundle spike interval (the A—H interval).
         c. Disturbances of AV nodal conduction result in prolongation of the A—H interval.
      4. His bundle
         a. There is no surface representation of His bundle activation; it is *implied* by a succeeding QRS complex.
         b. On the intracardiac electrogram, careful positioning of an electrode can demonstrate a small deflection coincident with the activation of the His bundle.
         c. The time between the His bundle spike and the QRS complex is the H—V interval.
         d. The sum of A—H and H—V intervals equals the PR interval.

5. Bundle branches
    a. Depolarization of the right and left bundles produce the QRS complex on the surface ECG.
    b. Defects of bundle branch conduction have been discussed on Day 3.

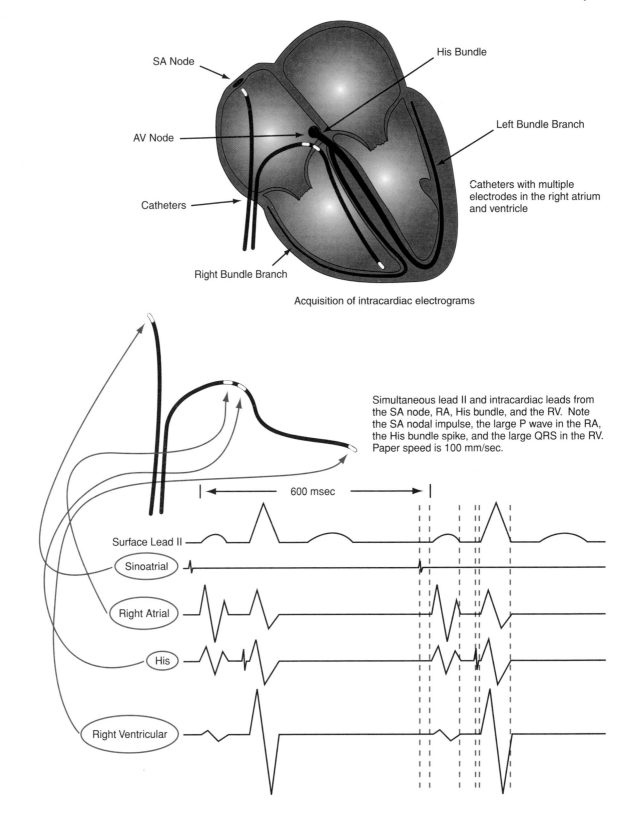

Acquisition of intracardiac electrograms

Simultaneous lead II and intracardiac leads from the SA node, RA, His bundle, and the RV. Note the SA nodal impulse, the large P wave in the RA, the His bundle spike, and the large QRS in the RV. Paper speed is 100 mm/sec.

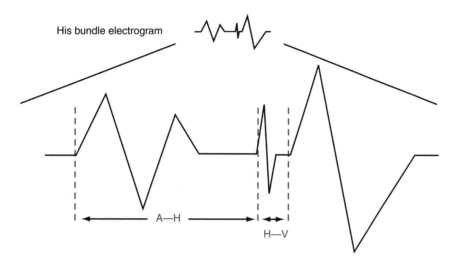

His bundle electrogram

II. AV conduction abnormalities

    A. First degree AV block

        1. In first degree AV block, the PR interval is > 200 ms.

        2. The PR interval is dependent on heart rate, so that at very slow rates, a PR interval > 200 may be normal.

        3. First degree AV block is almost always due to a prolongation of the A—H interval.

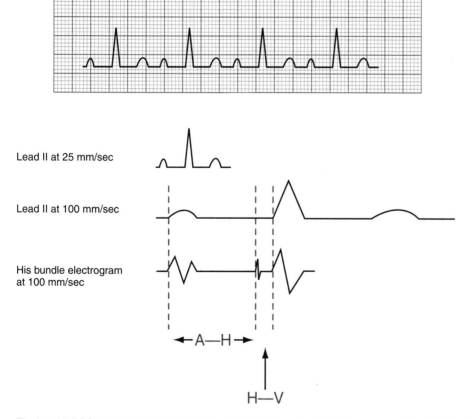

The Lead II ECG shows sinus rhythm with a very long PR interval of 280 msec, consistent with first degree AV block. The His bundle electrogram shows a prolongation of the A—H interval with a normal H—V interval. This finding is typical of delay in the AV node itself.

III. Second degree AV block

    A. Type I (Wenckebach)

        1. In second degree AV block type I, there is progressive prolongation of the PR interval until there is a dropped QRS complex.

        2. The Wenckebach phenomenon usually produces group beating of the QRS complexes.

        3. In the His bundle electrogram, there is progressive prolongation of the A—H interval until there is no His spike produced.

        4. The H—V interval is usually normal.

Lead II

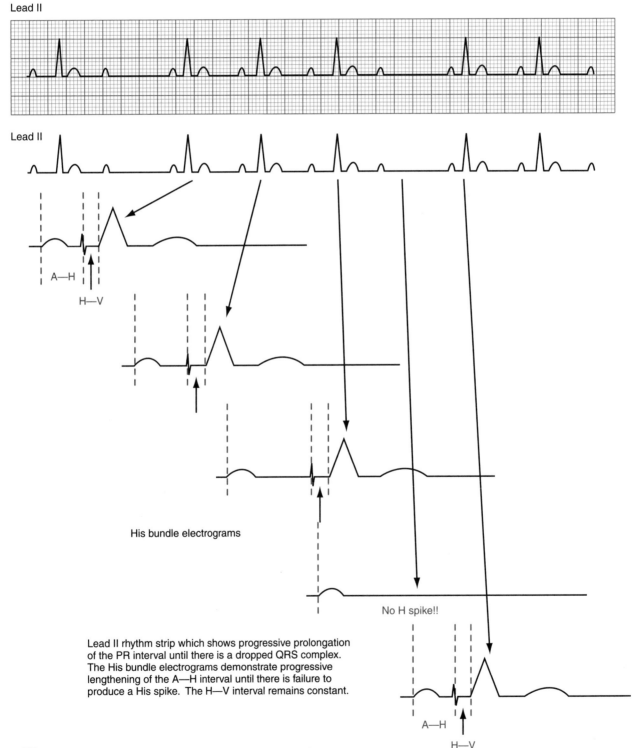

Lead II

A—H

H—V

His bundle electrograms

No H spike!!

Lead II rhythm strip which shows progressive prolongation
of the PR interval until there is a dropped QRS complex.
The His bundle electrograms demonstrate progressive
lengthening of the A—H interval until there is failure to
produce a His spike. The H—V interval remains constant.

A—H

H—V

B.   Second degree AV block type II
1.   In second degree AV block type II, there are regular P waves with an occasional loss of the QRS complex.
2.   The PR interval does not change before the conducted beats.
3.   On the His bundle electrogram, this type of block is usually associated with an intermittent failure of H—V conduction.

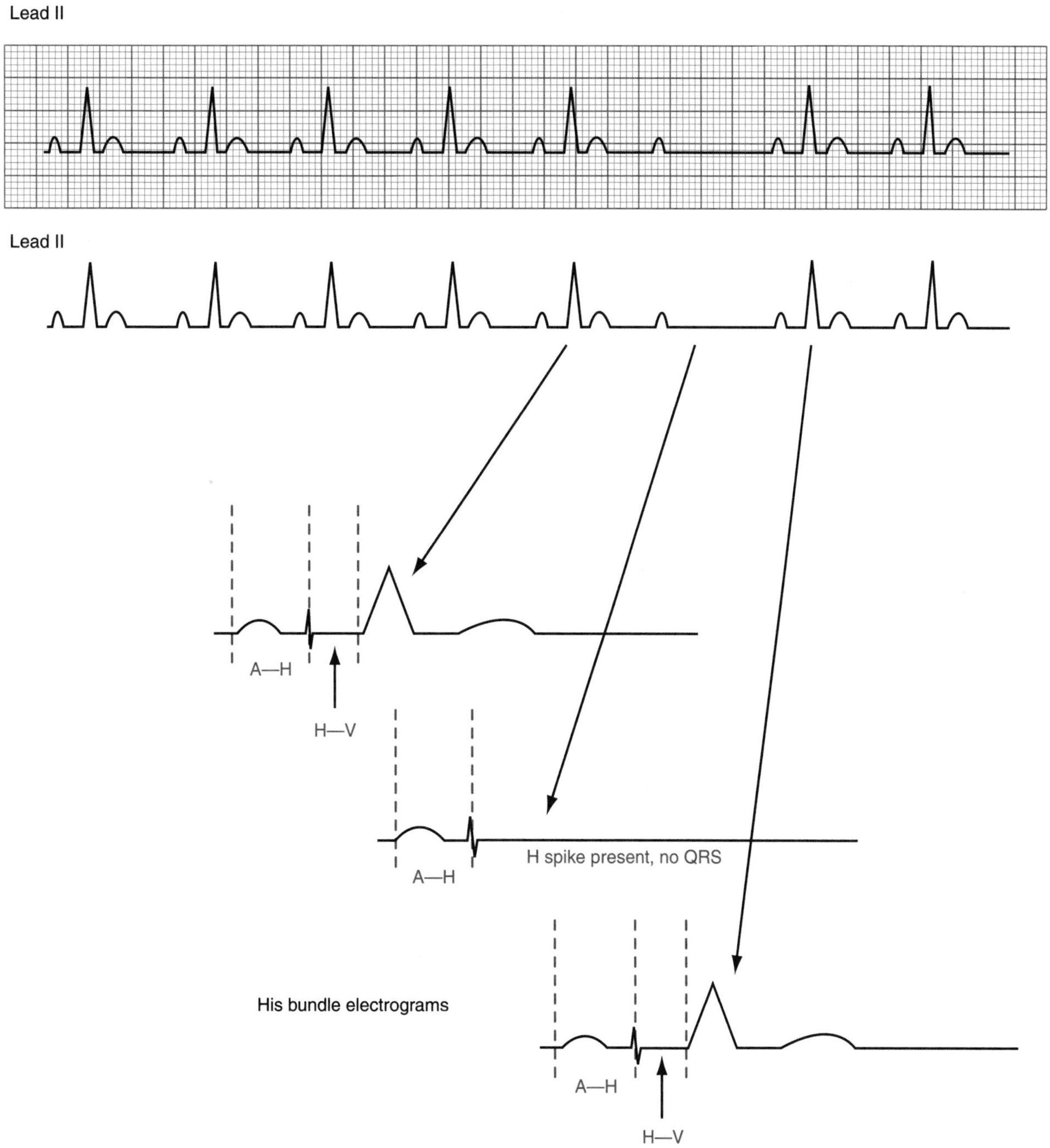

Lead II

Lead II

A—H

H—V

A—H

H spike present, no QRS

His bundle electrograms

A—H

H—V

Lead II rhythm strip which shows a single dropped QRS, with no change in the PR intervals of the conducted beats. The His bundle electrograms demonstrate a slightly prolonged H—V interval and a sudden failure to conduct to the ventricle. The A—H interval remains constant.

IV. Third degree AV block

    A. In third degree AV block, there is complete failure of conduction from the atria to the ventricles.

    B. The atrial rate is always faster than the ventricular rate.

    C. The escape rhythm may arise from the junctional area, in which case its rate will typically be 40–60, or it may arise from a ventricular focus with a rate of 20–40.

    D. Junctional escape rhythms have a narrow QRS complex (unless there is an accompanying bundle branch block), but ventricular rhythms will be wide (QRS > 120 msec).

    E. Third degree block is one form of A-V dissociation (see later in this chapter).

    F. There may be slight variation in the P-P intervals, with the P waves which surround a QRS complex being slightly closer together than those which do not (ventriculophasic sinus arrhythmia).

Lead II

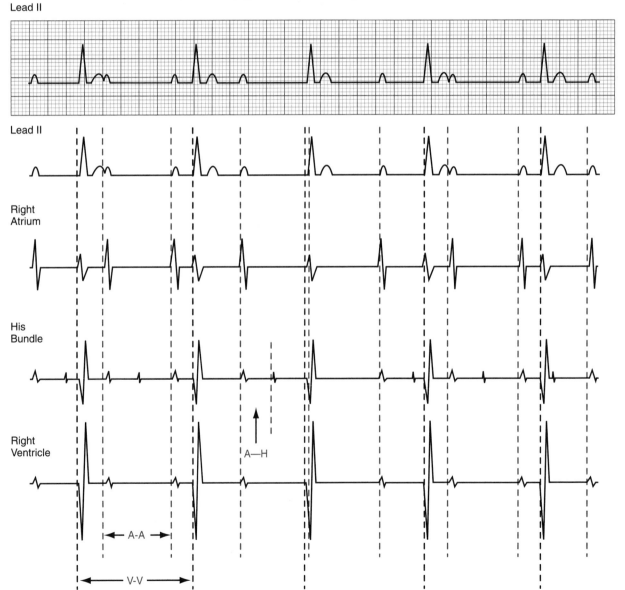

Surface Lead II and intracardiac electrograms in third degree AV block. Note the independent atrial (red dashed lines) and ventricular (black dashed lines) rhythms. In the His bundle electrogram, a His spike follows each atrial impulse (ie, the A—H interval is normal) but there is no succeeding ventricular depolarization. This represents complete failure of H—V conduction.

V. Summary of AV block

    A. First degree AV block is usually caused by a prolongation of the A—H interval.

    B. Second degree AV block type I (Wenckebach) is caused by progressive prolongation of the A—H interval.

    C. Second degree AV block type 2 is usually caused by an intermittent failure of H—V conduction.

    D. Third degree AV block is usually caused by a complete failure of H—V conduction.

    E. *In general,* A—H prolongation is a benign clinical event, while abnormalities of H—V conduction represent serious clinical situations that usually require permanent pacing.

First degree AV block Second degree AV block type I	}	Usually caused by delay of conduction in the AV node, resulting in A—H prolongation. This is typically a *benign* clinical situation.
Second degree AV block type II Third degree AV block	}	Usually caused by a block distal to the AV node, resulting in H—V conduction failure. This is usually a clinically unstable situation which requires permanent pacing.

VI. AV dissociation

    A. AV dissociation is present when there are independent atrial and ventricular rhythms.

    B. Types of AV dissociation
        1. By default
            a. In this case, there is a failure of conduction from a higher pacemaker, so that a lower pacemaker takes over.
            b. Third degree block is the principal example of this form of AV dissociation.
        2. By usurpation
            a. In this case, a lower pacemaker speeds up and usurps control from the higher pacemaker by virtue of being *faster.*
            b. Ventricular tachycardia (70% of which has AV dissociation) is an example of this form.

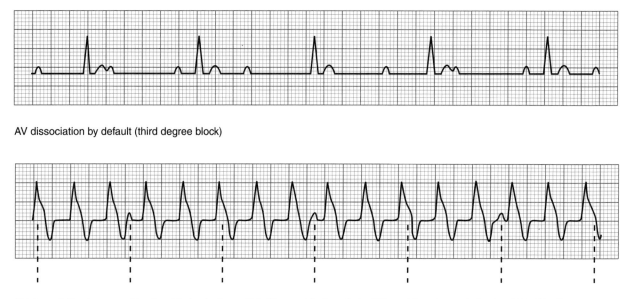

AV dissociation by default (third degree block)

AV dissociation by usurpation (ventricular tachycardia). The ventricular rate is 150, and the sinus rate is about 60. The P waves are indicated by the dashed lines.

VII. SA block

A. First degree, second degree type II, and third degree SA block cannot be identified on the surface ECG.

B. Second degree SA block type I produces an identifiable pattern of group beating on the ECG, with P waves of the same morphology and unchanging PR intervals.

In this cross section of the SA node, there is progressive delay of the SA nodal impulse until there is failure to "get out of" the node. This behavior produces second degree SA block type 1.

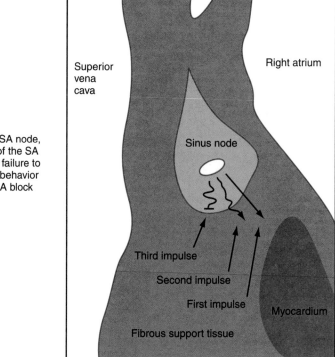

Lead II

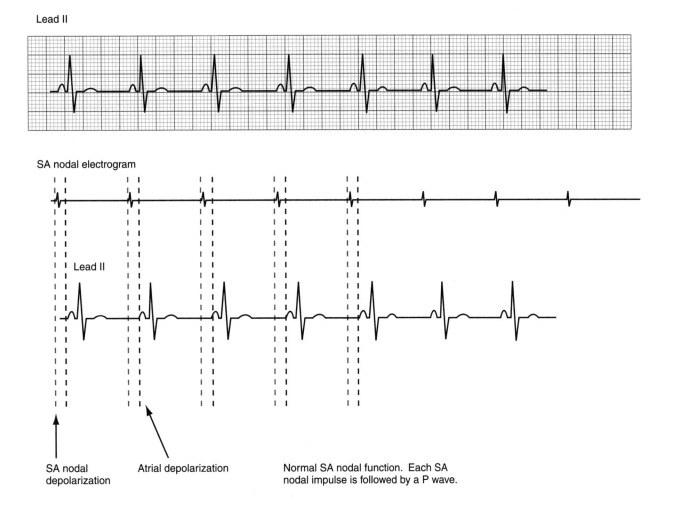

SA nodal electrogram

Lead II

SA nodal
depolarization

Atrial depolarization

Normal SA nodal function. Each SA
nodal impulse is followed by a P wave.

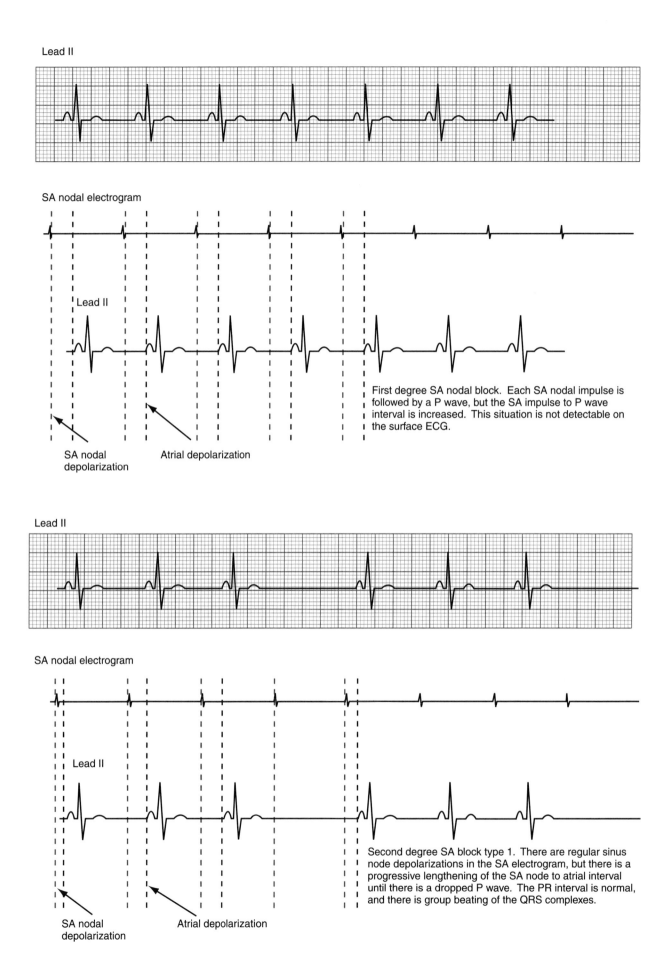

Lead II

SA nodal electrogram

Lead II

SA nodal
depolarization

Atrial depolarization

First degree SA nodal block. Each SA nodal impulse is followed by a P wave, but the SA impulse to P wave interval is increased. This situation is not detectable on the surface ECG.

Lead II

SA nodal electrogram

Lead II

SA nodal
depolarization

Atrial depolarization

Second degree SA block type 1. There are regular sinus node depolarizations in the SA electrogram, but there is a progressive lengthening of the SA node to atrial interval until there is a dropped P wave. The PR interval is normal, and there is group beating of the QRS complexes.

Lead II

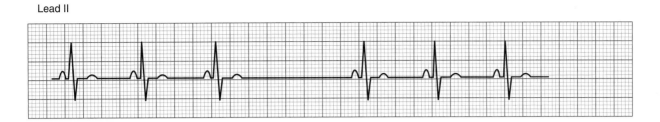

SA nodal electrogram

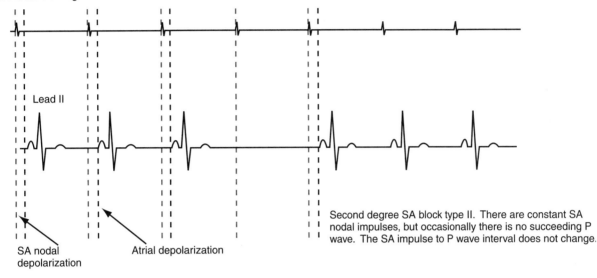

Lead II

SA nodal
depolarization

Atrial depolarization

Second degree SA block type II. There are constant SA nodal impulses, but occasionally there is no succeeding P wave. The SA impulse to P wave interval does not change.

Lead II

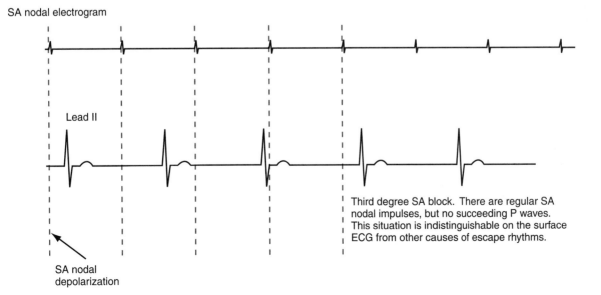

SA nodal electrogram

Lead II

SA nodal
depolarization

Third degree SA block. There are regular SA nodal impulses, but no succeeding P waves. This situation is indistinguishable on the surface ECG from other causes of escape rhythms.

THE GROUP BEATING TREE

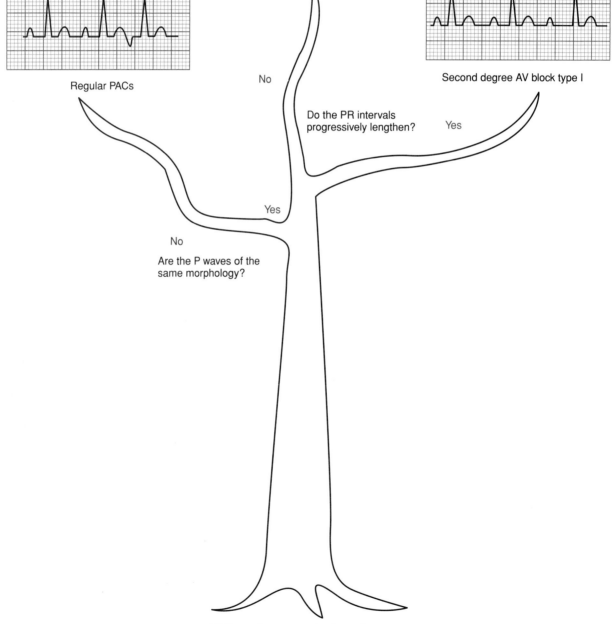
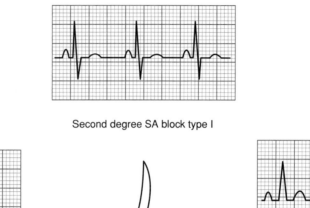

Second degree SA block type I

Regular PACs

No

Do the PR intervals
progressively lengthen?

Yes

Second degree AV block type I

Yes

No

Are the P waves of the
same morphology?

QRS complexes occurring in regular groups

Day 4 ECG 1

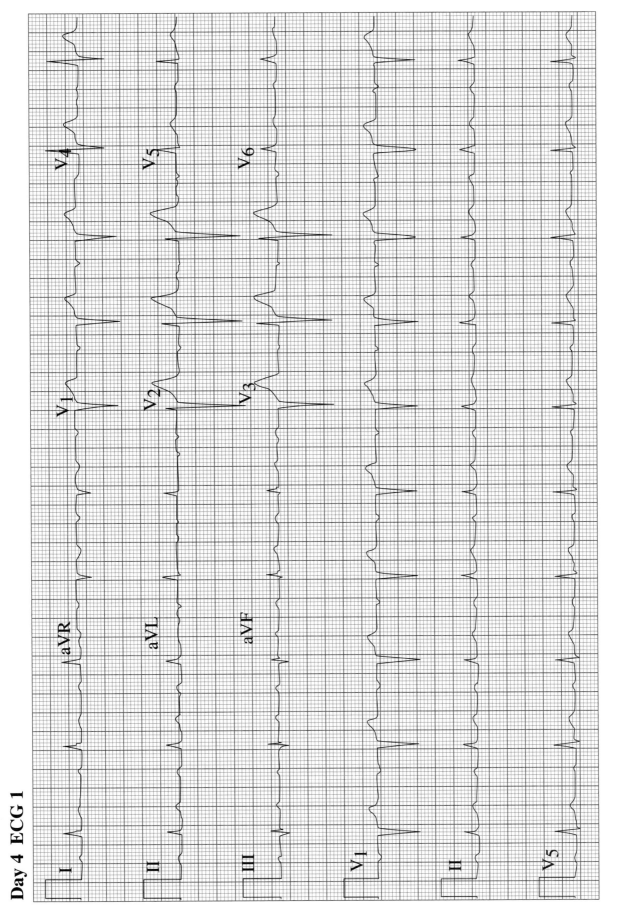

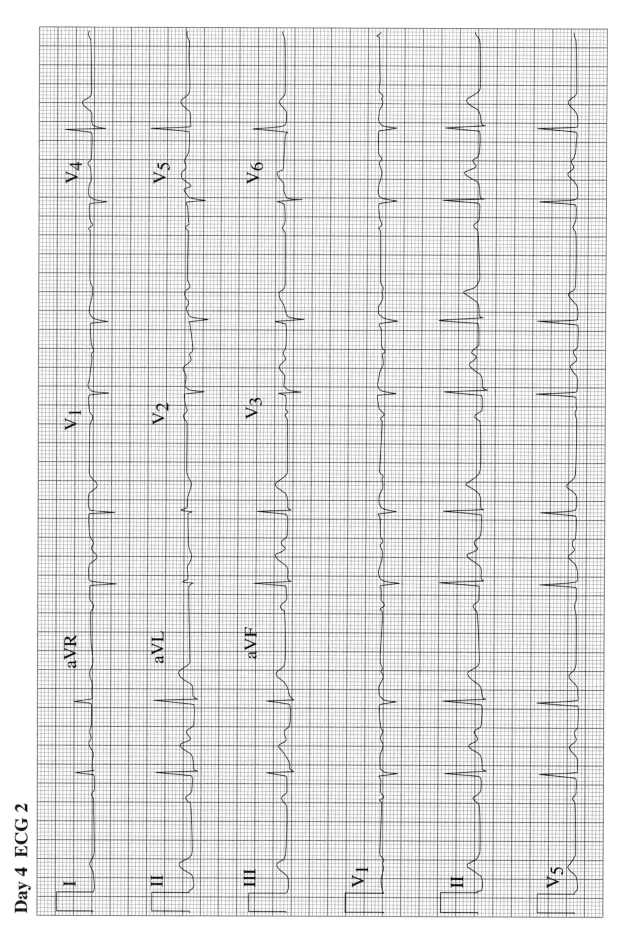

Day 4 ECG 3

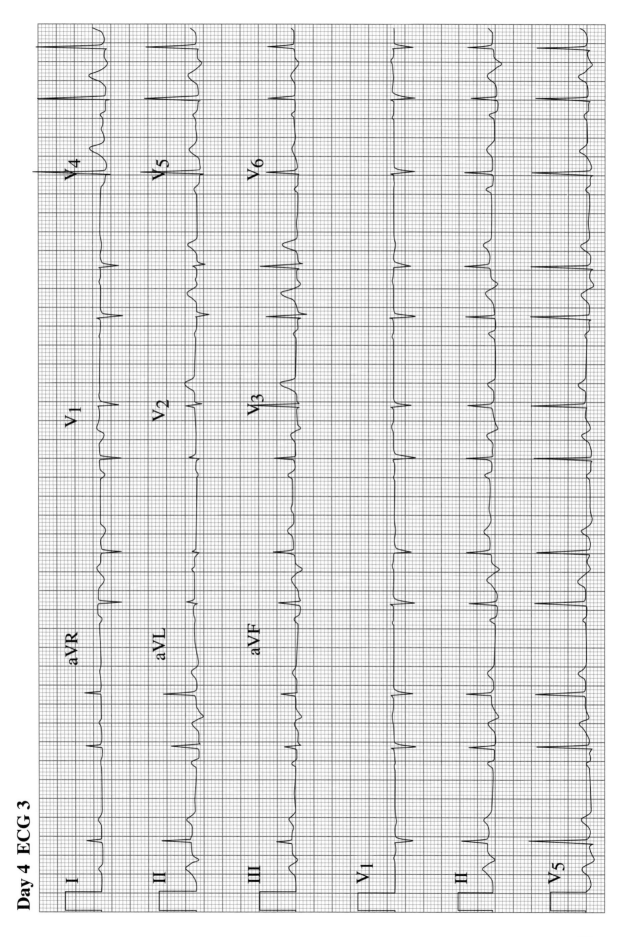

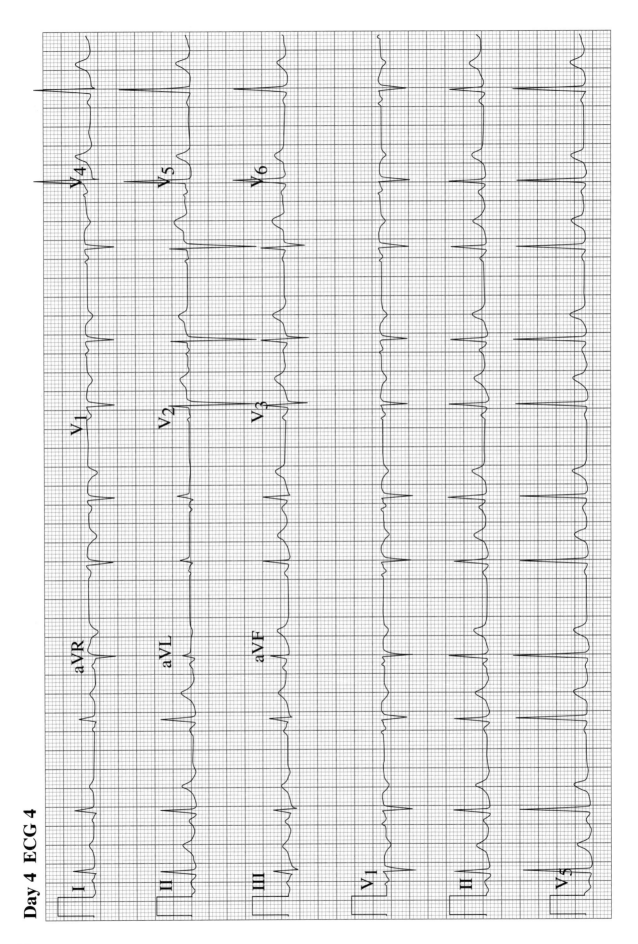

Day 4 ECG 5

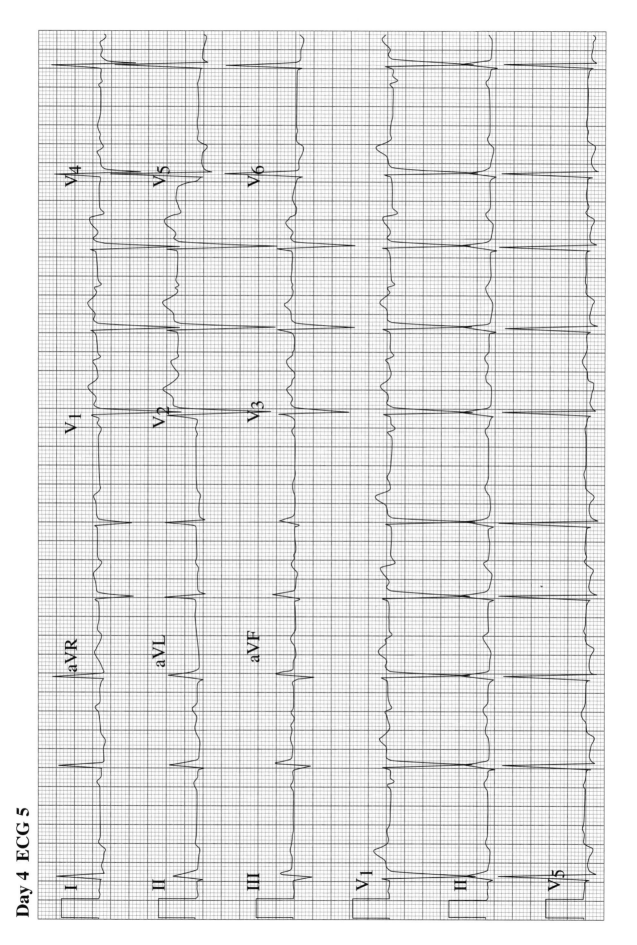

Day 4 ECG 6

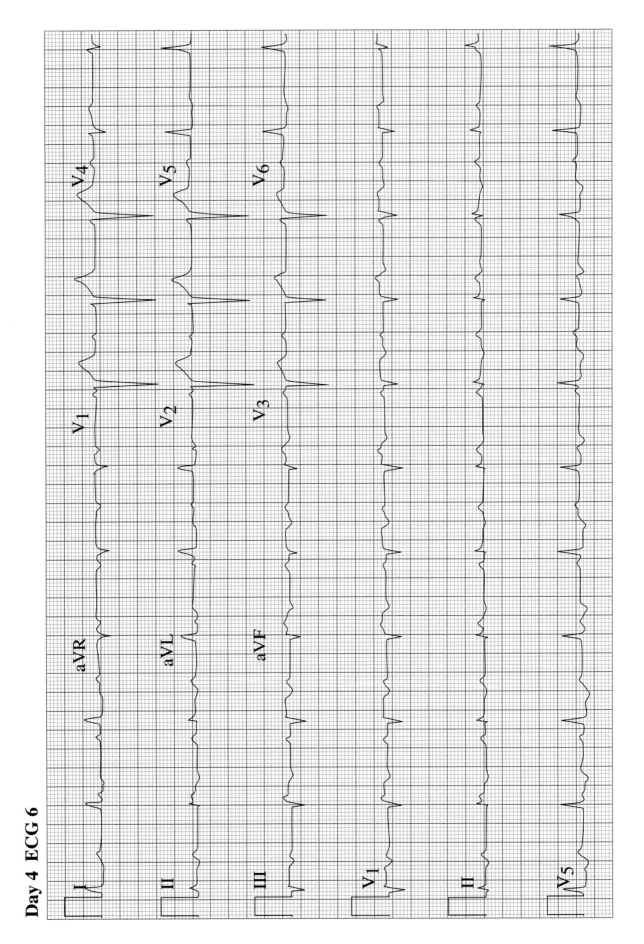

82

Day 4 ECG 7

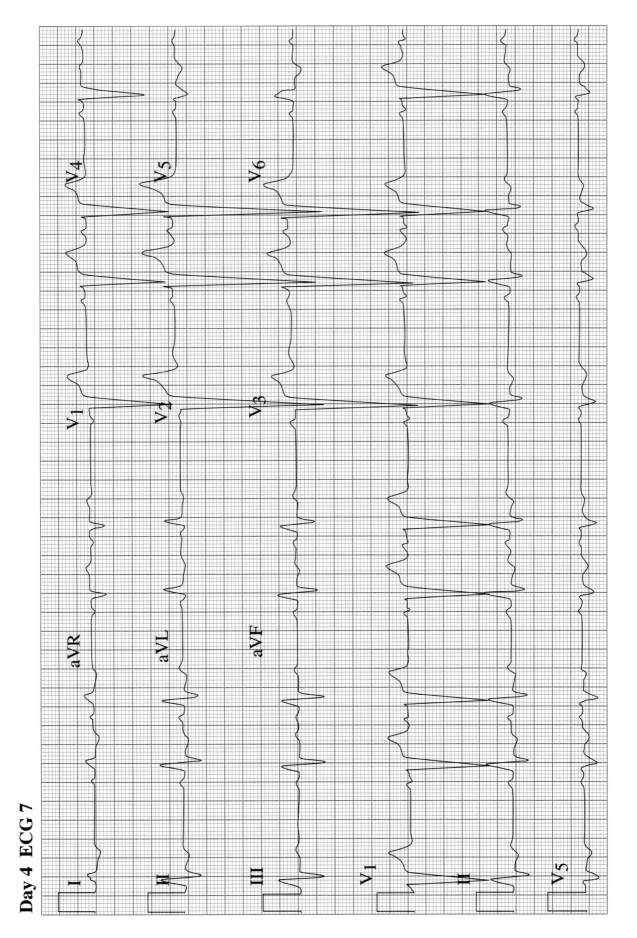

Day 4 ECG 8

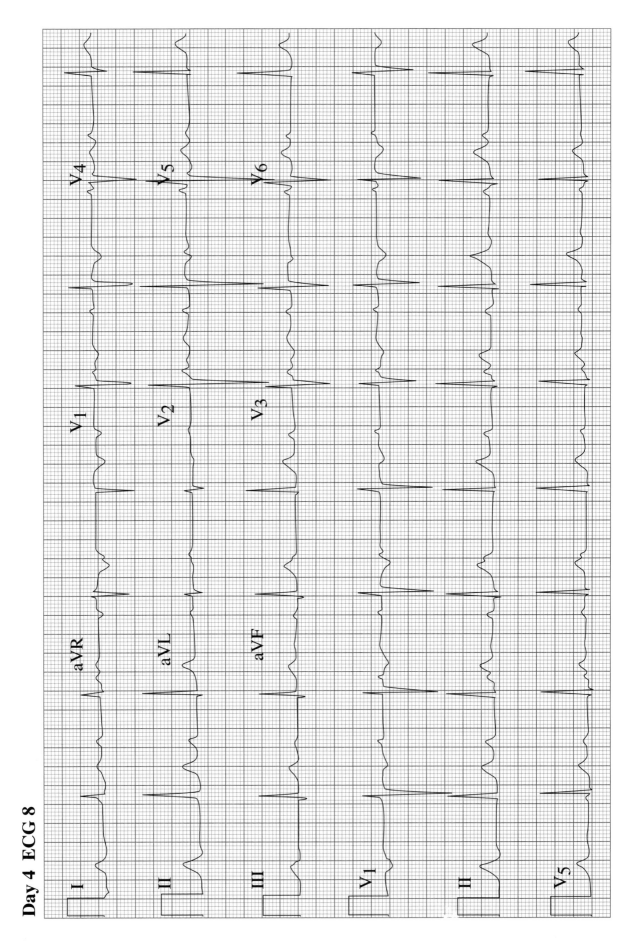

Day 4 ECG 9

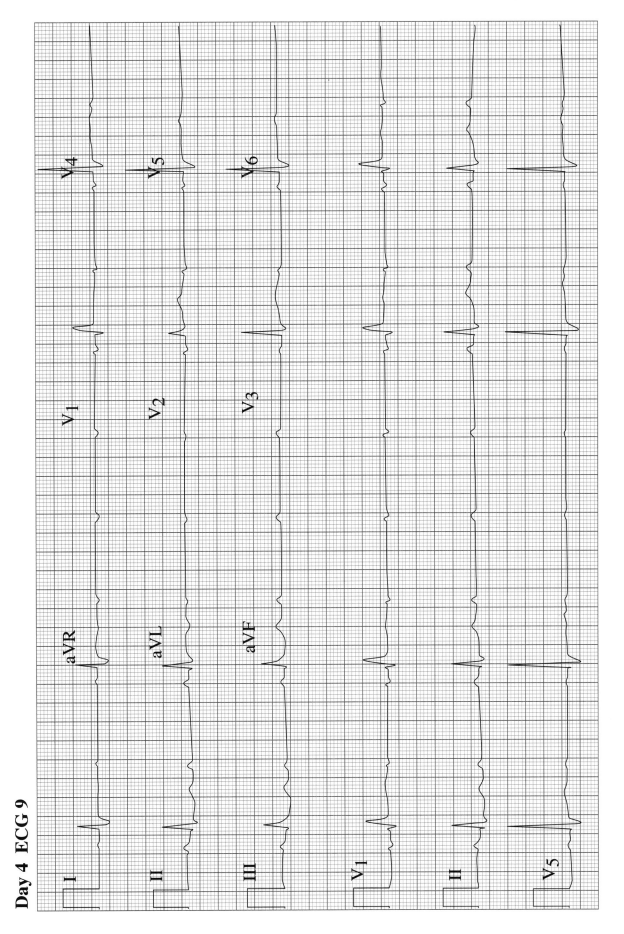

Day 4 ECG 10

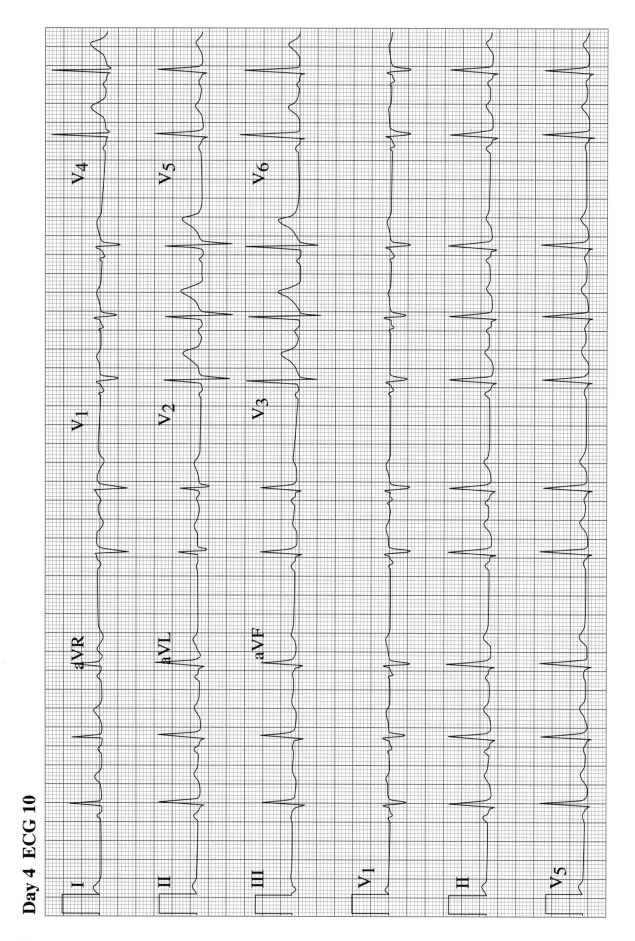

Day 4
ECG Interpretations and Discussion

Day 4 ECG 1
Normal sinus rhythm
First degree AV block

The PR interval is greater than 120 msec.

Day 4 ECG 2
Sinus rhythm
Second degree AV block type 1

There is group beating of the QRS complexes, the P waves have the same morphology, and there is progressive prolongation of the PR interval, indicating second degree AV block type 1.

Day 4 ECG 3
Sinus rhythm with regular premature atrial extrasystoles

There is group beating of the QRS complexes, but the second complex in each group is preceded by a P wave with a different morphology, indicating regular premature atrial extrasystoles.

Day 4 ECG 4
Sinus rhythm
Second degree SA block type 1

There is group beating of the QRS complexes, the P waves have the same morphology, and the PR interval is not prolonging, indicating second degree SA block type 1.

Day 4 ECG 5
Sinus rhythm
Second degree AV block type 1
Inferior MI, age undetermined
LVH with repolarization abnormalities

The P waves have a prominent terminal negativity in V_1, indicating left atrial abnormality. There is group beating of the QRS complexes, the P waves have the same morphology, and there is progressive prolongation of the PR interval, indicating second degree AV block type 1. There are Q waves in II, III, and aVF, indicating an inferior MI. There are voltage criteria for left ventricular hypertrophy in the precordial leads and ST and T wave changes consistent with repolarization abnormalities.

Day 4 ECG 6
> Sinus rhythm
> Third degree AV block
> Accelerated junctional escape rhythm
> Inferior MI, probably acute
> Possible anterior MI, age undetermined

There are independent sinus and junctional rhythms indicating third degree AV block. The escape rhythm is junctional because of its normal QRS duration, but the rate is faster than a typical junctional rate (40–60). There is ST segment elevation and Q waves in II, III, and aVF, indicating an acute inferior MI. There is also a Q wave in V_3 and delayed precordial transition, suggesting a previous anterior MI. AV block is a fairly common complication of an acute inferior MI, since the AV nodal artery is supplied by the right coronary artery 85% of the time, and occlusion of the right coronary is responsible for most inferior infarctions. AV block with an inferior MI is generally a benign clinical event.

Day 4 ECG 7
> Sinus rhythm
> Second degree SA block type 1
> Left bundle branch block

There is group beating of the QRS complexes, the P waves have the same morphology, and the PR interval is not prolonging, indicating second degree SA block type 1. The QRS complexes are greater than 120 msec, the intrinsicoid deflection time is prolonged in I and V_6, and there is a monophasic R wave in those leads, consistent with a left bundle branch block.

Day 4 ECG 8
> Sinus rhythm
> Third degree AV block
> Junctional escape rhythm

There are independent sinus and junctional rhythms indicating third degree AV block. The escape rhythm is junctional because of its normal QRS duration. This patient is a 23-year-old female with congenital complete heart block.

Day 4 ECG 9
> Sinus rhythm
> Second degree AV block type 2
> Right bundle branch block

There is sinus rhythm with frequent and consecutive dropped QRS complexes, indicating second degree AV block type 2. The QRS complexes are greater than 120 msec, there is a delayed intrinsicoid deflection time in V_1, an RSR' pattern in V_1, and wide S waves in I and V_6, all consistent with right bundle branch block.

Day 4 ECG 10
> Sinus rhythm
> Second degree SA block type 1

There is group beating of the QRS complexes, the P waves have the same morphology, and the PR interval is not prolonging, indicating second degree SA block type 1.

Day 5

Ischemia and Infarction

I. The ST segment and T wave in ischemia

    A. There are over 100 identified causes of ST segment and T wave changes, so the diagnosis of ischemia and infarction frequently requires comparison with previous ECGs and correlation with the clinical presentation and laboratory data.

    B. Myocardial ischemia produces a range of changes in the ST segment and T wave, depending on the severity of ischemia and the timing of the ECG.

    C. The specificity of ST segment and T wave changes is decreased in patients with resting abnormalities, particularly LBBB and LVH.

    D. The specificity of the ST segment for ischemia is also dependent on its morphology.

    E. In exercise stress testing, 1 mm or more of horizontal or downsloping ST segment depression 80 msec from the J point is considered an ischemic response.

Forms of ST segment depression

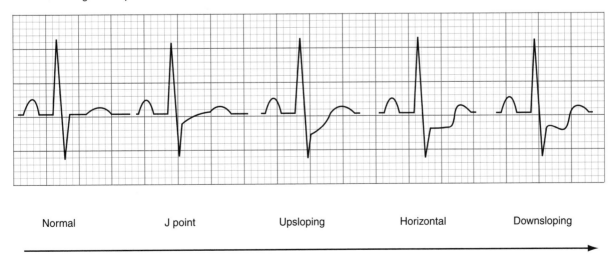

Normal   J point   Upsloping   Horizontal   Downsloping

Increasing specificity for ischemia

89

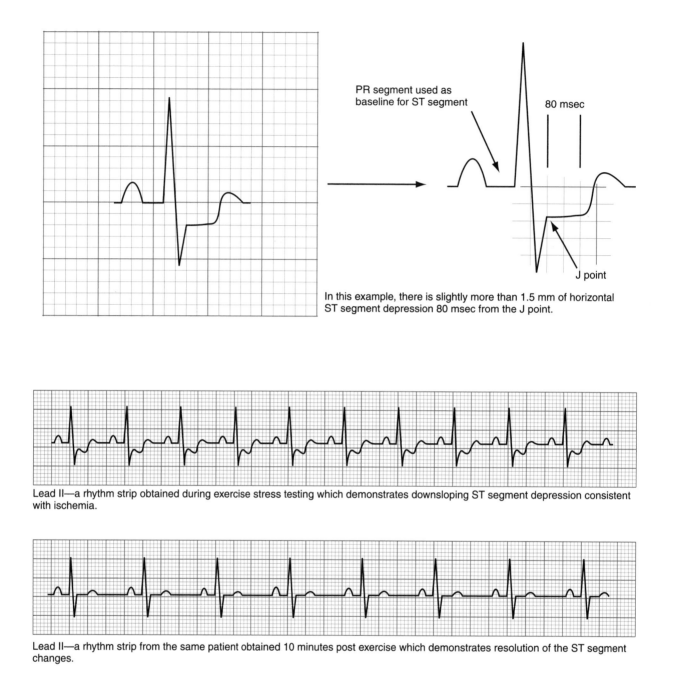

PR segment used as baseline for ST segment

80 msec

J point

In this example, there is slightly more than 1.5 mm of horizontal ST segment depression 80 msec from the J point.

Lead II—a rhythm strip obtained during exercise stress testing which demonstrates downsloping ST segment depression consistent with ischemia.

Lead II—a rhythm strip from the same patient obtained 10 minutes post exercise which demonstrates resolution of the ST segment changes.

II. Myocardial infarction

    A. ECG patterns in infarction
        1. A zone of ischemia typically produces ST segment depression.
        2. A zone of injury produces ST segment elevation.
        3. A zone of infarction produces a large Q wave in the QRS complex.

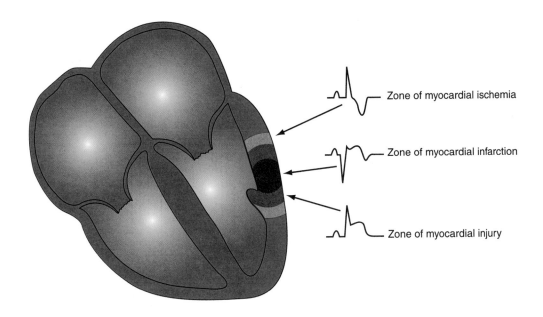

Zone of myocardial ischemia

Zone of myocardial infarction

Zone of myocardial injury

B. Genesis of the Q wave in infarction
    1. The normal situation
        a. For example, in Lead I, the QRS complex begins with a small Q wave because left ventricular depolarization begins in the septum and the electrical forces are directed away from Lead I.
        b. The small Q wave is rapidly succeeded by forces directed inferiorally and laterally, resulting in a large R wave in Lead I.

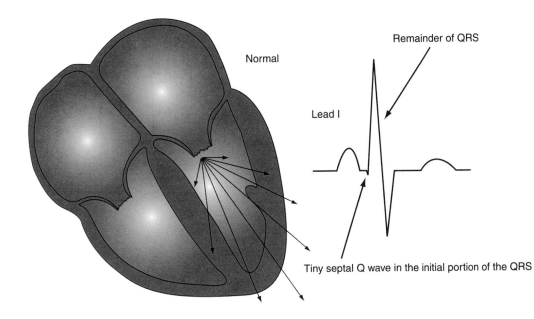

Normal

Remainder of QRS

Lead I

Tiny septal Q wave in the initial portion of the QRS

2. The infarct situation
    a. If there is a lateral myocardial infarction, however, the electrical
        vectors in the lateral direction are lost, the forces directed medially
        are unbalanced, a large Q wave results in Lead I.

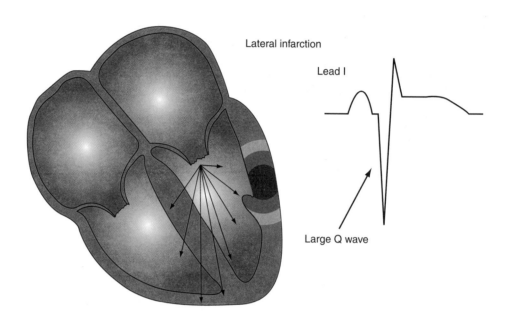

Lateral infarction

Lead I

Large Q wave

III. The time course of myocardial and ECG changes during infarction

First and second days

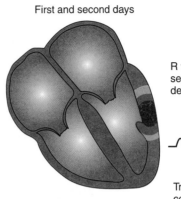

R wave nearly gone, ST segment elevation decreased, T wave inverted

Transmural infarction nearly complete, some injury may persist at borders

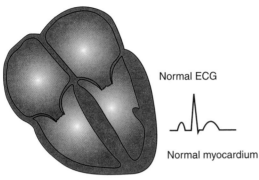

Normal ECG

Normal myocardium

Onset and first several hours

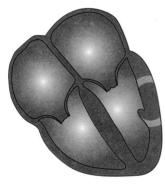

Normal R wave, peaked ST segment and T wave

Subendocardial injury and myocardial ischemia, no infarction yet

After 2 or 3 days

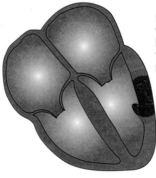

No R wave, deep Q wave, ST segment back to baseline, T wave inversion persists

Transmural infarction

First day

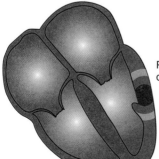

R wave amplitude diminishes

Ischemia and injury extend to epicardial surface, subendocardial muscle dying

After several weeks or months

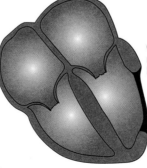

Q waves persist, small R wave may return, T wave inversion lessens

Infarcted myocardium

IV. Anatomical and ECG locations of MI

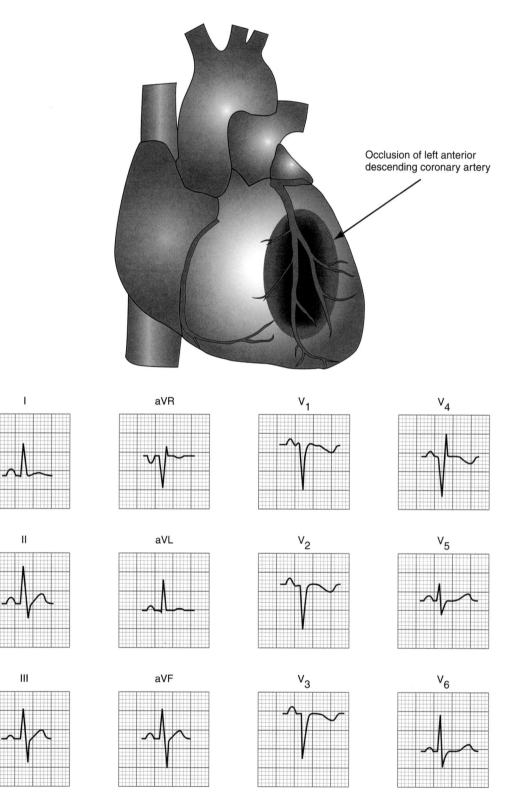

ECG demonstrating an anterior myocardial infarction with prominent Q waves in V_1–V_4.

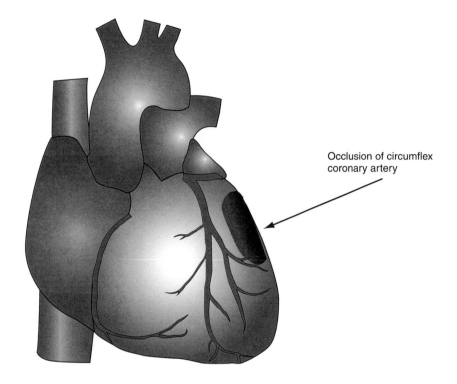

Lateral infarct

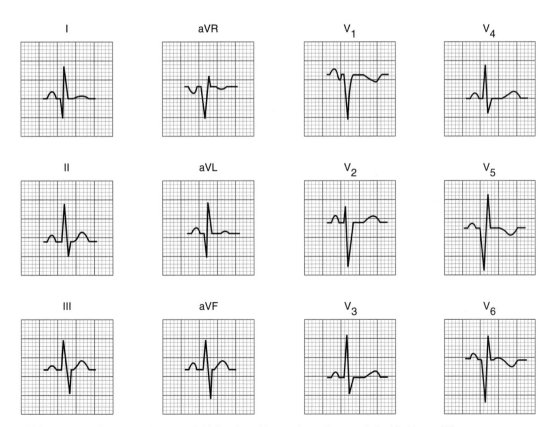

ECG demonstrating a lateral myocardial infarction with prominent Q waves in I, aVL, V_5, and V_6.

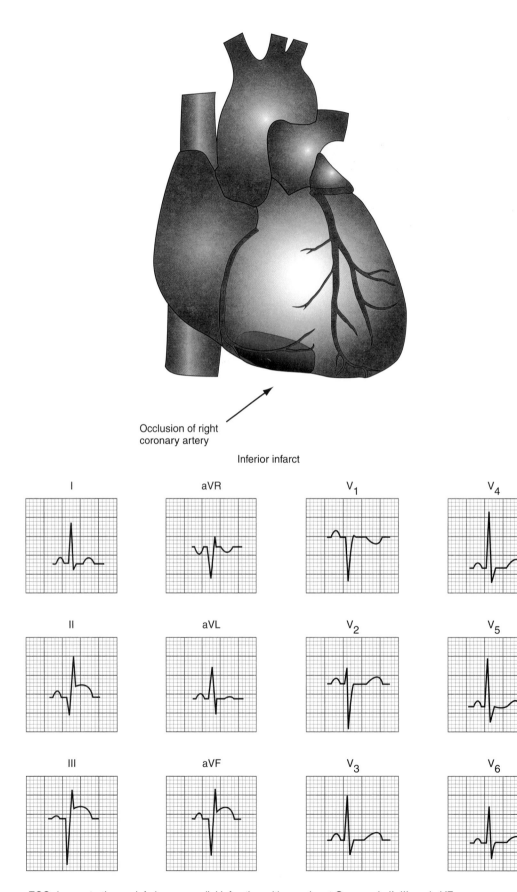

Occlusion of right
coronary artery

Inferior infarct

ECG demonstrating an inferior myocardial infarction with prominent Q waves in II, III, and aVF.

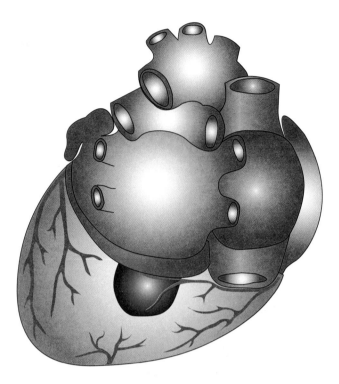

Posterior infarct

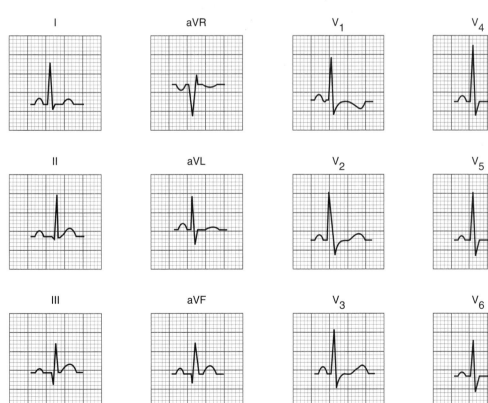

ECG demonstrating a posterior myocardial infarction with a prominent R wave in V_1, as well as a probable inferior MI with small Q waves in III and aVF.

V.   Non-Q wave MI (NQMI)

A.   About half of the 750,000 MIs which occur annually in the U.S. do not develop new Q waves.

B.   A variety of ECG findings are typical, including ST segment and T wave changes.

C.   About 20% of NQMIs have no localizable ST or T wave changes.

D.   Anatomically, NQMI is frequently associated with patchy subendocardial necrosis.

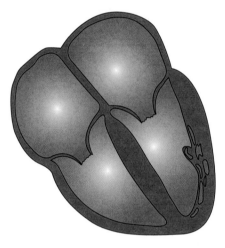

Non-Q wave infarct

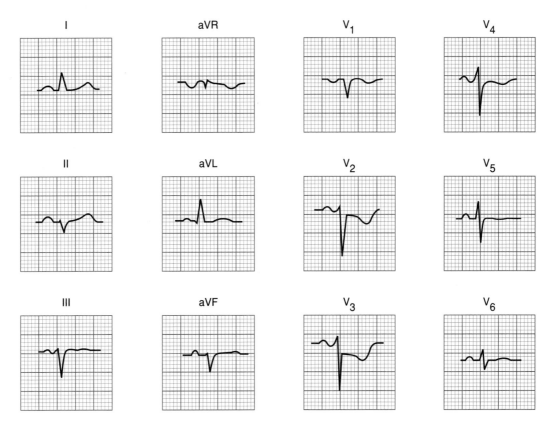

I   aVR   V₁   V₄

II   aVL   V₂   V₅

III   aVF   V₃   V₆

ECG demonstrating diffuse anterolateral ST segment depression and T wave inversion. Cardiac enzymes were positive for a CK-MB rise, indicating a non-Q wave myocardial infarction.

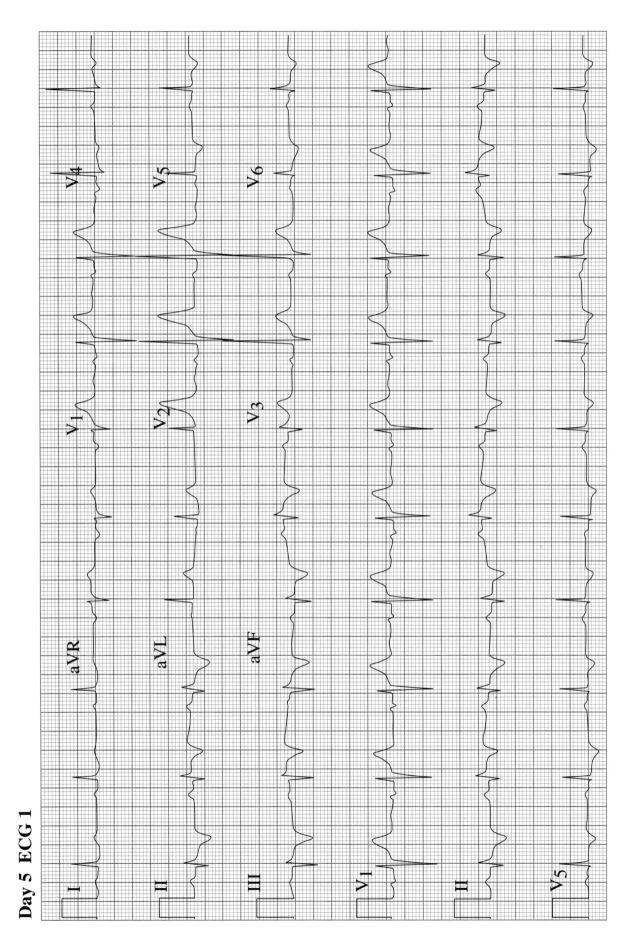

Day 5 ECG 2

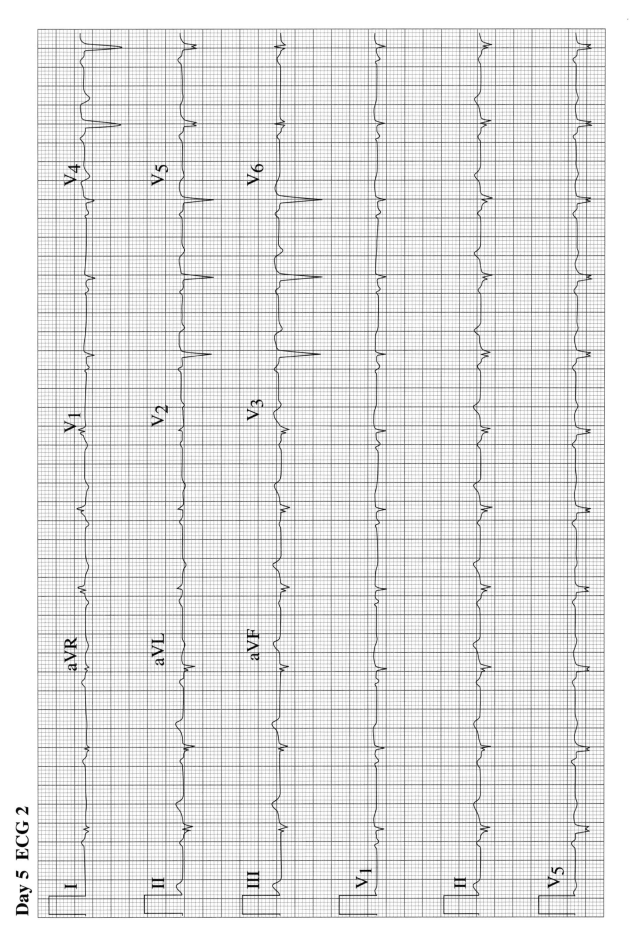

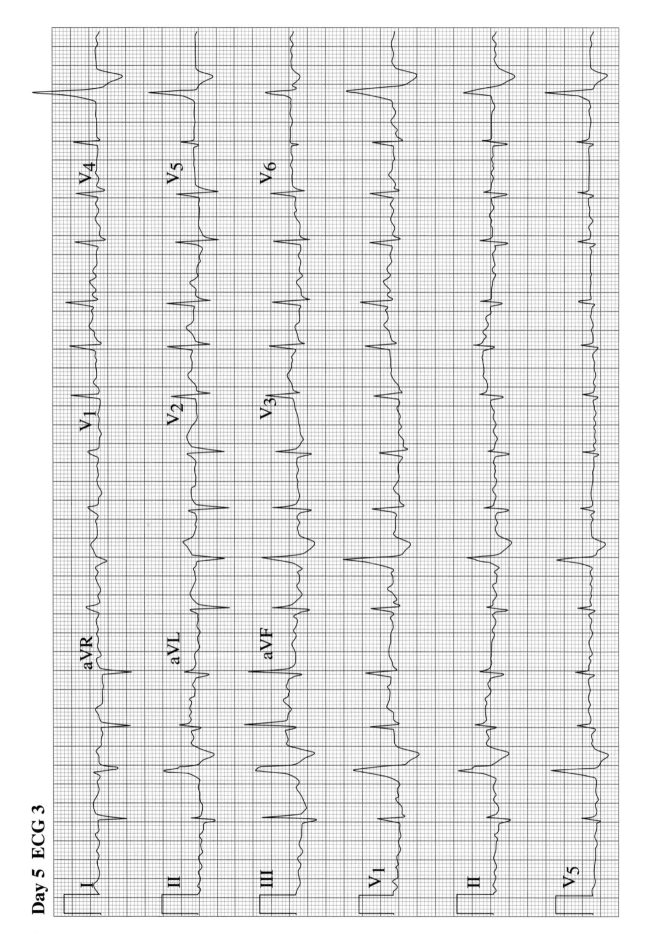

Day 5 ECG 4

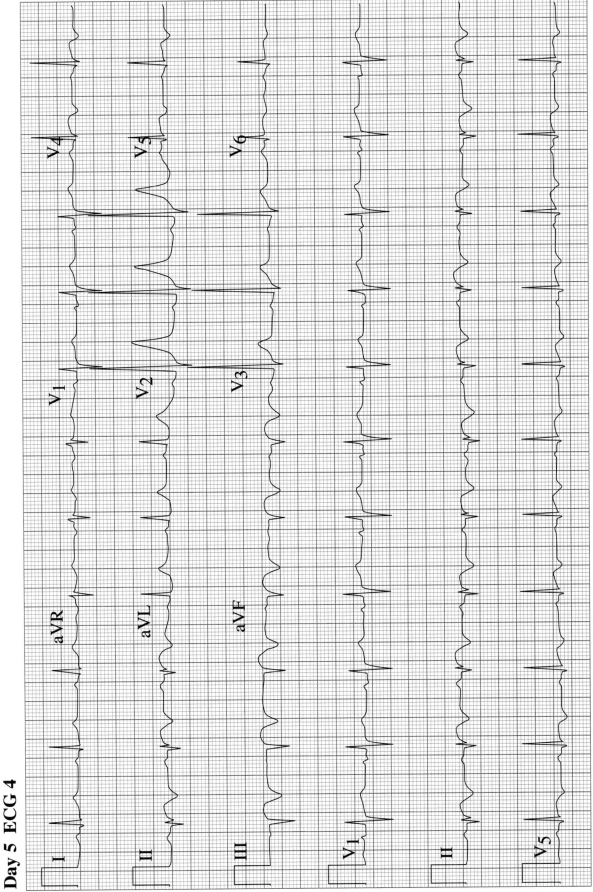

Day 5 ECG 5

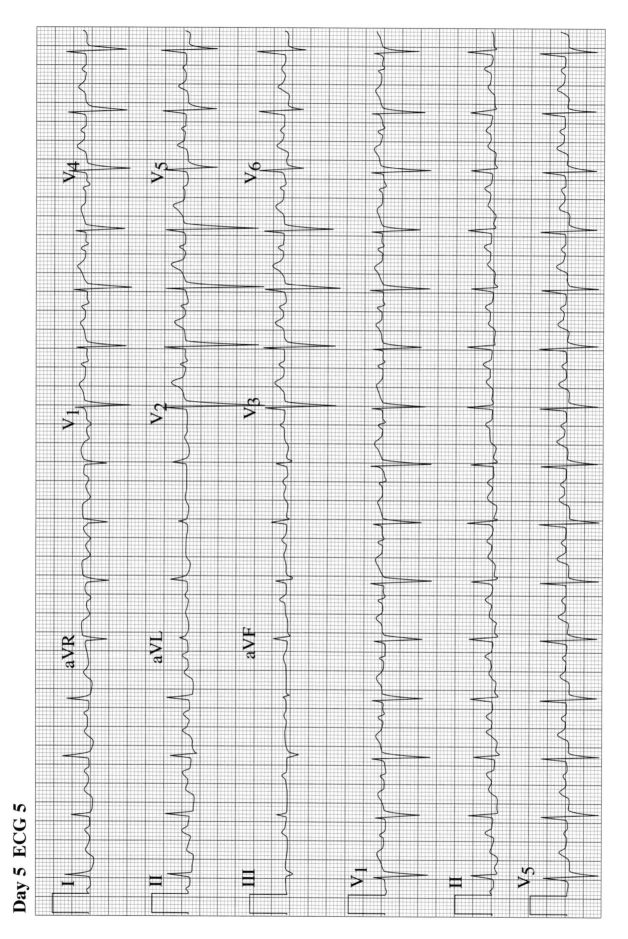

Day 5 ECG 6

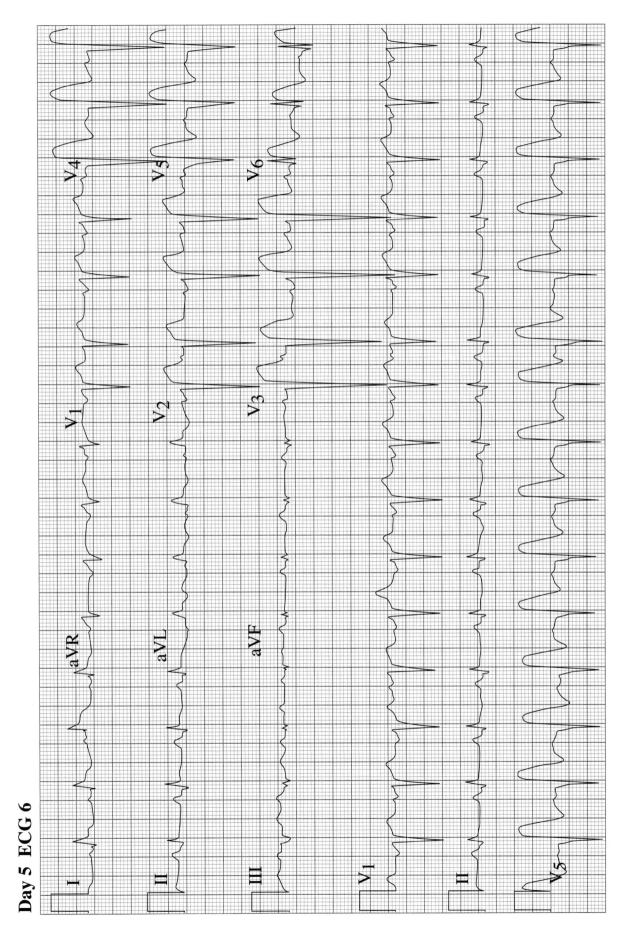

Day 5 ECG 7

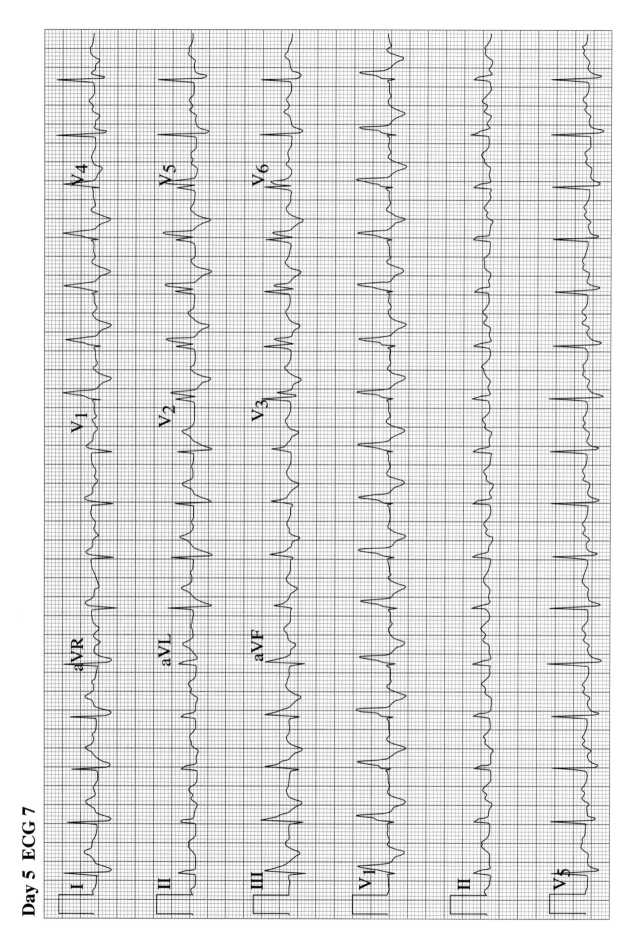

Day 5 ECG 8

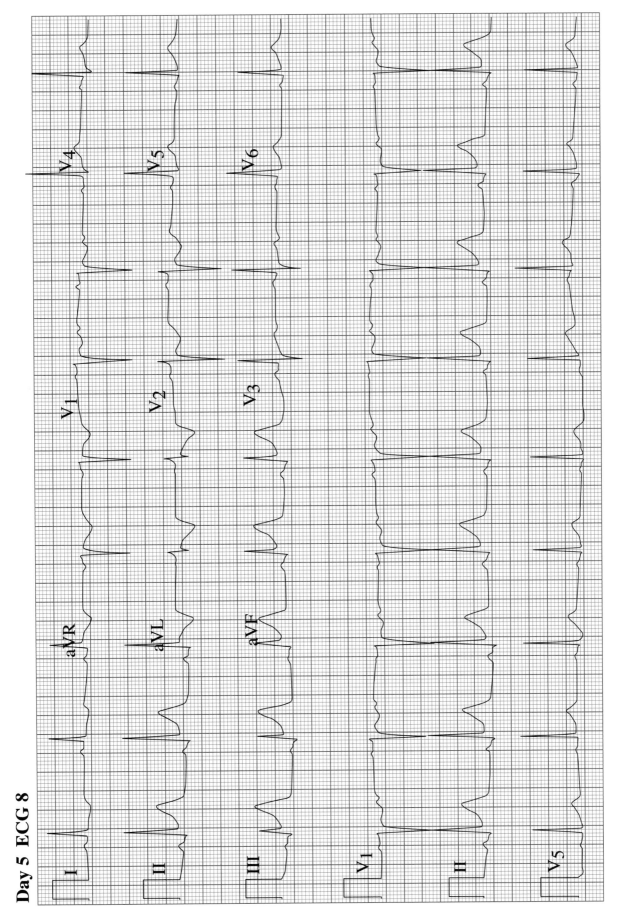

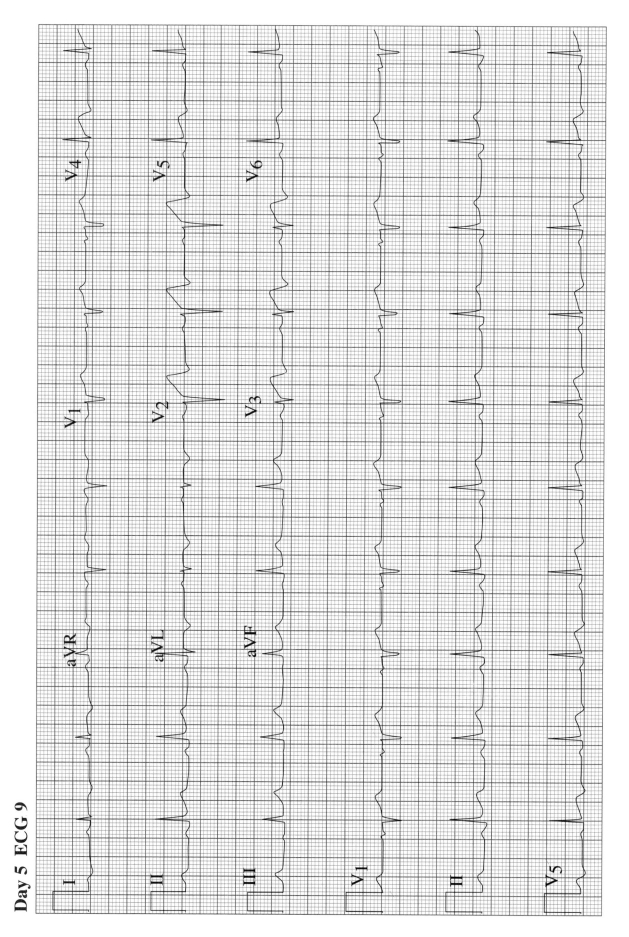

Day 5 ECG 9

Day 5 ECG 10

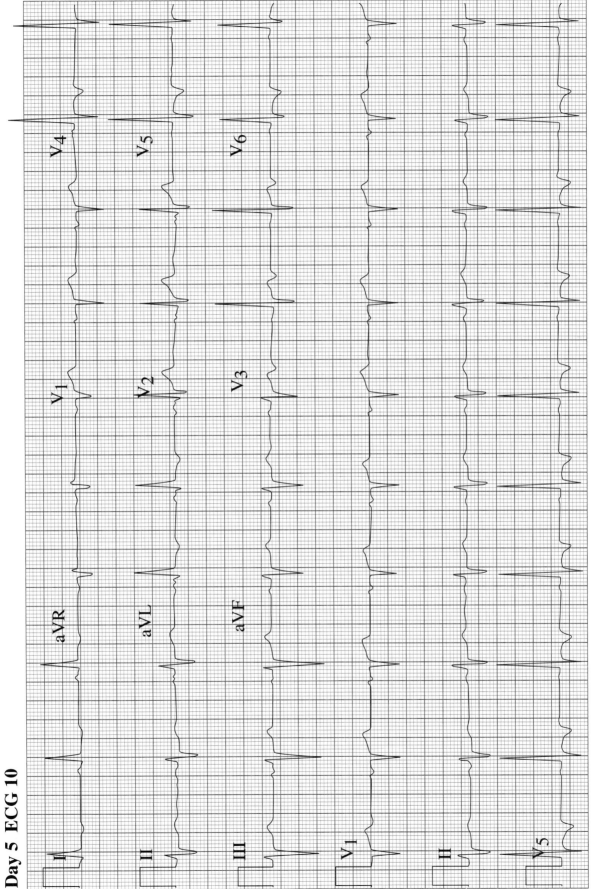

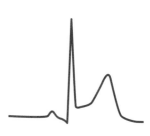

Day 5
ECG Interpretations and Discussion

Day 5 ECG 1
Normal sinus rhythm
Inferoposterior MI, probably recent

There are Q waves, some residual ST segment elevation, and T wave inversion in II, III, and aVF, as well as prominent R waves in V_1 and V_2, indicating a recent inferoposterior MI.

Day 5 ECG 2
Normal sinus rhythm
Anterolateral MI, age undetermined
Inferior MI, age undetermined
Low voltage

There are Q waves and some ST segment elevation in V_1–V_5, consistent with an anterior MI. The clinical event in this patient was 3 months prior to this ECG, so the residual ST segment elevation may represent a ventricular aneurysm. There is loss of R waves in the lateral leads, suggesting involvement in that area. There are small Q waves and very small R waves in II, III, and aVF, consistent with a previous inferior MI.

Day 5 ECG 3
Atrial fibrillation with rapid ventricular response
Ventricular extrasystoles
Right axis deviation
Lateral MI, age undetermined
Inferoposterior MI, age undetermined

There is an irregular baseline with irregular QRS complexes, indicating atrial fibrillation. The ventricular rate is greater than 100. There are wide QRS complexes consistent with ventricular extrasystoles. The QRS complex is downward in I and upright in aVF, indicating right axis deviation. There are Q waves in I, V_5, and V_6, indicating a lateral MI. There are Q waves in II, III, and aVF and tall R waves in V_1, indicating an inferoposterior MI. The right axis deviation is due to the lateral MI.

Day 5 ECG 4
Normal sinus rhythm
Left axis deviation
Recent inferoposterior MI
ST and T wave changes; consider lateral ischemia

The QRS complex is upright in I, and downward in aVF and II, indicating left axis deviation. There are Q waves, ST segment elevation, and T wave inversion in II, III, and aVF, as well as tall R waves in V_1 and V_2, consistent with a recent inferoposterior MI. There are ST segment and T wave changes extending into the lateral leads, suggesting ischemia surrounding the infarct.

Day 5 ECG 5
> Normal sinus rhythm
> ST segment depression; consider inferolateral ischemia

There is downsloping ST segment depression in the inferior and lateral leads, suggesting ischemia.

Day 5 ECG 6
> Sinus tachycardia
> Acute anterolateral MI
> Probable inferior MI, age undetermined

There are Q waves and hyperacute ST segment elevation in the anterior and lateral leads, indicating an acute anterolateral MI. There are small Q waves and tiny R waves in the inferior leads, suggesting a previous inferior MI.

Day 5 ECG 7
> Sinus tachycardia
> First degree AV block
> Right bundle branch block
> Probable inferior MI, age undetermined

The PR interval is greater than 200 msec. The QRS complexes are greater than 120 msec, there is a delayed intrinsicoid deflection time in V1, an RSR′ pattern in V_1, and wide S waves in I and V_6, all consistent with right bundle branch block. There are rather small Q waves in II, III, and aVF, suggesting a previous inferior MI.

Day 5 ECG 8
> Sinus bradycardia
> Acute inferior MI

The heart rate is less than 60. There is hyperacute ST segment elevation in the inferior leads, indicating an acute inferior MI. There are no Q waves yet, consistent with a very recent onset of ischemia. The ST segment depression in V_1 and V_2 may represent a posterior extension of the infarct.

Day 5 ECG 9
> Normal sinus rhythm
> Acute anterior MI

There is hyperacute ST segment elevation in the anterior leads, indicating an acute anterior MI.

Day 5 ECG 10
> Normal sinus rhythm
> Left axis deviation
> Left ventricular hypertrophy with repolarization abnormalities

The QRS complex is upright in I, and downward in aVF and II, indicating left axis deviation. There are voltage criteria for left ventricular hypertrophy. There is ST segment depression and T wave inversion in several leads which could ordinarily be attributed to repolarization abnormalities with left ventricular hypertrophy, but in this case the changes are more pronounced than in a recent ECG, suggesting an ischemic component.

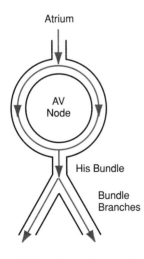

Day 6

Mechanisms of Arrhythmias

I. Narrow versus wide complex arrhythmias

   A. All narrow QRS complex arrhythmias originate above the His bundle and are called supraventricular.

   B. Supraventricular arrhythmias can have wide QRS complexes if there is a concomitant intraventricular conduction defect.

   C. The differential diagnosis is the subject of Day 8.

II. Reentry—a disorder of impulse transmission. All arrhythmias should be considered reentrant until proven otherwise, as reentry is responsible for 90% of arrhythmias.

   A. Mechanisms of reentry
      1. Reentry requires:
         a. At least two conduction pathways
         b. Variable block in one of the pathways

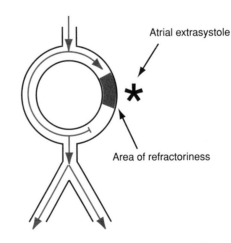

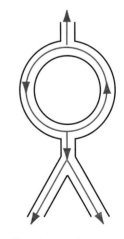

Normal AV nodal conduction using both intranodal pathways

An atrial extrasystole blocks conduction in one limb of the AV node, blocking conduction in that pathway.

The normal impulse travels retrograde up the blocked limb. When it arrives, the limb has recovered and allows transmission, thus perpetuating the arrhythmia. The atria are depolarized from below.

2. If two pathways have similar conduction velocities, the electrical impulses will merge distally and no arrhythmia will occur (see figure below).

3. If an event (eg, an atrial extrasystole) occurs at the right time and place to make one of the two pathways refractory, the impulse will be blocked in that limb.

4. If the impulse from the other limb travels back up the blocked limb, it may find the previously refractory area able to conduct.

5. If the impulse reaches the initial branch point of the two pathways before the next normal impulse arrives from above, the arrhythmia can perpetuate itself.

B. Properties of reentrant arrhythmias
    1. Reentrant arrhythmias start and stop abruptly (paroxysmally).
    2. They are usually initiated by a premature beat.
    3. The reentrant arrhythmias which have a discreet reentrant pathway (atrial flutter, PSVT, most VT) are very regular.
    4. Reentrant arrhythmias can be terminated by any mechanism which makes some part of the reentrant pathway refractory, including vagal maneuvers (PSVT), chest thump (VT), medications which slow conduction (most reentrant arrhythmias) or electrocardioversion (all reentrant arrhythmias).

III. The major reentrant arrhythmias

A. Atrial fibrillation—the most commonly encountered arrhythmias
    1. Mechanisms and causes
        a. Probably due to multiple reentrant wave fronts in the atrium.
        b. Requires a certain amount of atrial tissue to be present to sustain fibrillation (an important concept in therapeutic approaches).
        c. Atrial pressure overload (the most common cause is elevated ventricular diastolic pressure from coronary artery disease, hypertension, or chronic lung disease) is responsible for the vast majority of cases.

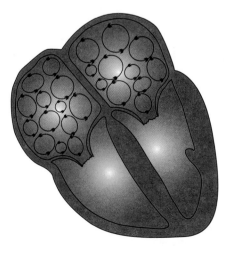

Typical multiple reentrant pathways in atrial fibrillation

Lead V$_1$—atrial fibrillation with slow ventricular response

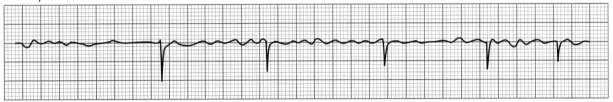

Lead V$_1$—atrial fibrillation with slow ventricular response

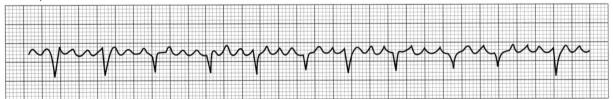

Lead V$_1$—atrial fibrillation

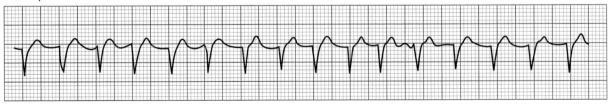

Lead V$_1$—atrial fibrillation with rapid ventricular response and RBBB

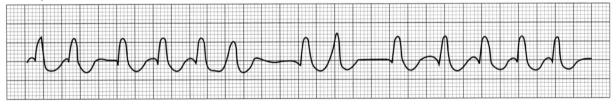

Lead V$_1$—atrial fibrillation with rapid ventricular response

Lead V$_1$—atrial fibrillation with rapid ventricular response

2. Heart rate
   a. The multiple reentrant wave fronts combine to have an atrial rate of 400–600.
   b. The ventricular response is irregular.
3. ECG morphology
   a. The baseline varies from coarse, irregular fibrillatory waves to virtually flat.
   b. The QRS complexes are narrow unless there is an IVCD.
4. Response to vagal maneuvers
   a. Vagal maneuvers do not affect the atrial fibrillation itself.
   b. The ventricular response is irregularly slowed.

B. Atrial flutter
   1. Mechanisms and causes
      a. Most examples are due to reentry.
      b. The common reentry pathway is counterclockwise in the right atrium and the interatrial septum.
      c. Atrial pressure overload (from similar conditions that cause atrial fibrillation) is responsible for the vast majority of cases.
   2. Heart rate
      a. The atrial rate is 250–350, more commonly 280–320, with a median of 300.
      b. Patients receiving antiarrhythmic therapy (eg, with quinidine, sotalol, or amiodarone) may have slower flutter rates.
      c. The ventricular response is usually a whole even number division of the atrial rate (2:1, 4:1, 8:1), although alternating 2:1/4:1 or variable ventricular responses are encountered.
      d. Every absolutely regular supraventricular tachycardia with a rate of 150 is atrial flutter with 2:1 block until proven otherwise.
   3. ECG morphology
      a. The baseline usually demonstrates distinct, extremely regular sawtooth flutter waves in Leads II, III, aVF, or V_1.
      b. The QRS complexes are narrow unless there is an IVCD.

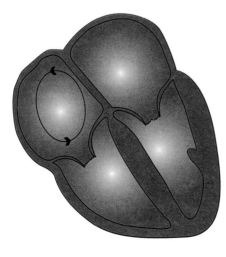

Typical reentrant pathway in atrial flutter with a counterclockwise pathway in the right atrium

Lead V₁—atrial flutter with 2:1 block. Note that at this ventricular rate, it is difficult to discern the flutter waves.

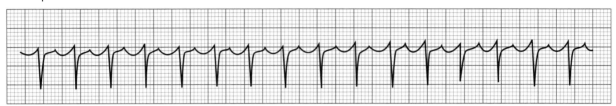

Lead V₁—the same patient with atrial flutter and 4:1 block

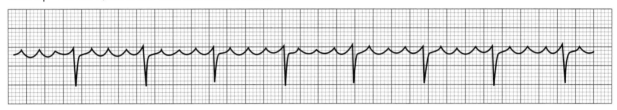

Lead II—atrial flutter with alternating 2:1 and 4:1 block

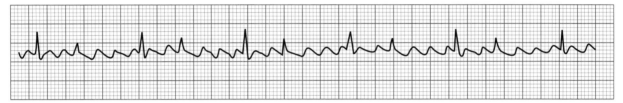

Lead II—atrial flutter with variable block

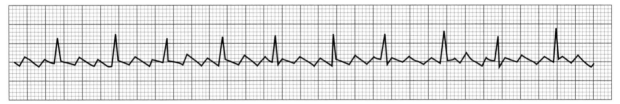

Lead II—an amazing case of atrial flutter with complete heart block and one ventricular escape complex

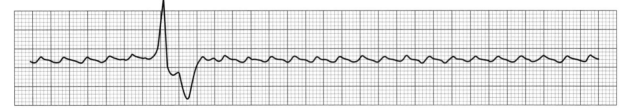

4. Response to vagal maneuvers
    a. Vagal maneuvers do not affect the atrial flutter itself.
    b. The ventricular response is slowed in whole number divisions of the atrial rate.

C. Paroxysmal supraventricular tachycardia (PSVT)
    1. Mechanisms and causes
        a. Most examples are likely due to reentry.
        b. The commonest reentry pathway involves the AV node (70% of cases, and is then called AV nodal reentrant tachycardia [AVNRT]).
        c. The pathway may be intraatrial (not involving the AV node), or may utilize an accessory pathway as part of the reentrant loop (see Day 7).
        d. PSVT may occur in otherwise completely normal individuals, or may occur as a result of increased atrial pressure or because of the presence of an accessory pathway.
        e. In AVNRT, the inciting event is usually an atrial extrasystole which renders the fast or slow pathway in the AV node refractory, thus allowing reentry to occur (see figure below).
    2. Heart rate
        a. The PSVT rate is typically 120–220.
        b. The ventricular rate is usually the same as the atrial rate.
    3. ECG morphology
        a. In the common form of AVNRT, the impulse travels down the slow pathway and up the fast pathway; thus the P wave is buried within the QRS complex.

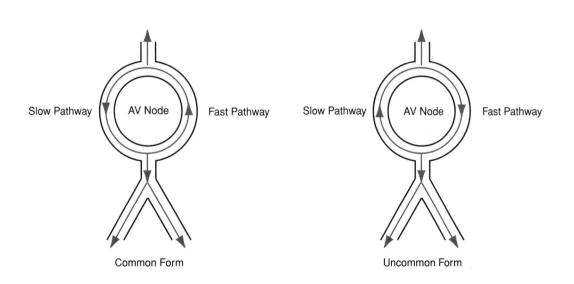

Lead II—the common form of AVNRT (PSVT). Note the retrograde P waves following the QRS complexes.

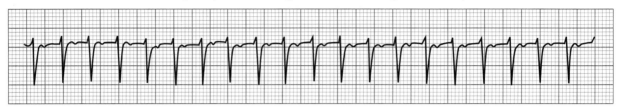

Lead II—the common form of AVNRT (PSVT). Note the retrograde P waves immediately following the QRS complexes.

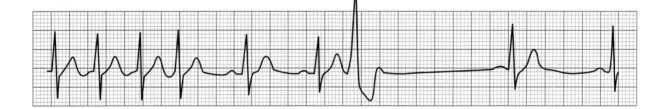

Lead V$_5$—PSVT which stops suddenly and reverts to normal sinus rhythm under the influence of carotid massage

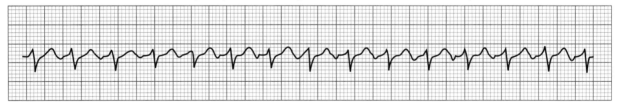

Lead II—the uncommon form of AVNRT (PSVT). Note the retrograde P waves far from the QRS complexes.

b. In the uncommon form, the impulse travels down the fast pathway and up the slow pathway; thus the P wave is between the QRS complexes.

c. The P wave axis is almost always abnormal because the atria are depolarized from below, not from the SA node.

4. Response to vagal maneuvers—vagal maneuvers cause increased AV block and may terminate the arrhythmia.

D. Ventricular tachycardia (VT)
1. Mechanisms and causes
   a. Most examples are due to reentry (90%).
   b. The reentry pathway frequently involves the edges of a previously infarcted area of myocardium, but also may be present in any condition which causes a myocardial abnormality.
   c. VT rarely occurs in healthy individuals.
2. Heart rate
   a. The VT rate is typically 120–220.
   b. The atrial rhythm may remain the same as it was prior to the development of VT (70% of the time, in which case there is AV dissociation), or there may be retrograde conduction to the atrium (30%, no AV dissociation).
3. ECG morphology
   a. VT demonstrates a wide QRS morphology.
   b. For a discussion of the differentiation of wide QRS tachycardias, see Day 8.
4. Response to vagal maneuvers—vagal maneuvers rarely have an effect on VT.

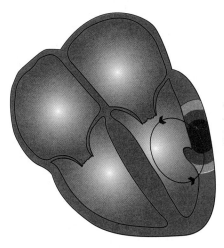

Typical reentrant pathway in ventricular tachycardia. The variable conduction produced by a myocardial infarction facilitates the reentry mechanism.

Lead II—wide QRS tachycardia consistent with VT

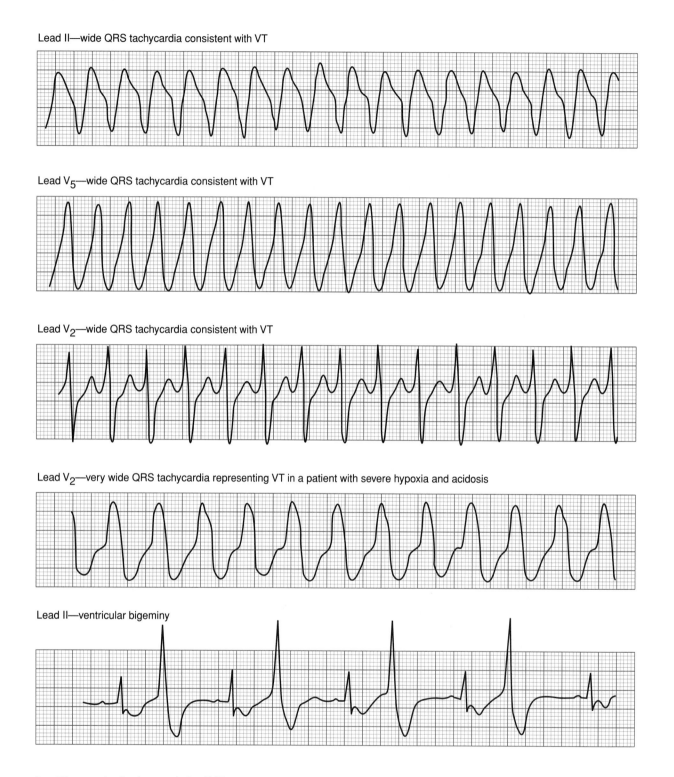

Lead V$_5$—wide QRS tachycardia consistent with VT

Lead V$_2$—wide QRS tachycardia consistent with VT

Lead V$_2$—very wide QRS tachycardia representing VT in a patient with severe hypoxia and acidosis

Lead II—ventricular bigeminy

Lead II—an episode of non-sustained VT

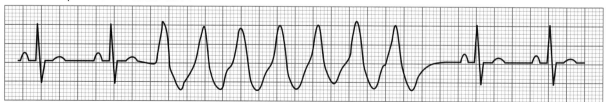

E. Ventricular fibrillation (VF)
1. Mechanisms and causes
a. VF probably represents multiple chaotic reentrant pathways involving the entire ventricular muscle.
b. VF occurs in patients with severe ischemia, hypoxia, metabolic abnormalities, etc.
c. VF is obviously rapidly fatal unless defibrillated.
2. ECG morphology—VF demonstrates an erratic baseline with no organized activity.

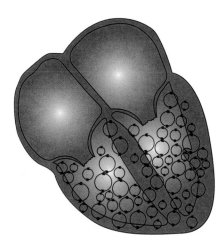

Multiple ventricular reentrant pathways in ventricular fibrillation

Lead II—disorganized baseline typical of VF

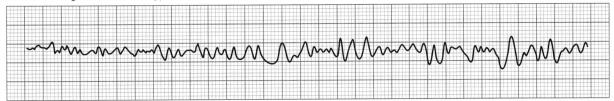

Summary of reentrant arrhythmias

ARRHYTHMIA	REENTRANT RATE	ECG DESCRIPTION	EFFECTS OF VAGAL MANEUVERS
Atrial Fibrillation	400–600	Irregular baseline, no regular P waves, irregular ventricular response	Slows ventricular response irregularly, no effect on atrial fibrillation
Atrial Flutter	250–350	Regular sawtooth P waves, regular ventricular response, usually even whole number divisions of atrial rate	Slows ventricular response in regular divisions of atrial rate, no effect on atrial flutter
PSVT	120–220	One inverted P wave for each QRS, P wave usually buried in QRS complex	May terminate the PSVT abruptly
VT	120–220	Wide QRS tachycardia (see Day 8)	No effect
VF	—	Irregular baseline with no organized ventricular activity	No effect

IV. Ectopy—a disorder of impulse formation. Only consider an ectopic source for an arrhythmia if no reentrant arrhythmia is plausible.

    A. Mechanisms of ectopic arrhythmias
       1. Ectopic arrhythmias require:
          a. Default—slowing of the normal dominant sinus pacemaker which allows a slower focus to take control, or
          b. Usurpation—an acceleration of a lower pacemaker which takes control by virtue of being faster than the sinus rate.
       2. Disorders of the sinus node, such as SA arrest, SA exit block, or excessive vagal tone may allow a lower focus to take control by default.
       3. A variety of factors, including digitalis toxicity, hypoxia, electrolyte disturbances, ischemia, or chronic lung disease may stimulate an ectopic focus to accelerate and usurp control from the SA node.

    B. Properties of ectopic arrhythmias
       1. Ectopic arrhythmias usually start and stop gradually (non-paroxysmally).
       2. They are not usually initiated by a premature beat.
       3. They may be somewhat irregular.
       4. They are not terminated by vagal maneuvers, although AV block may be increased.
       5. AV block of varying degrees is frequently present (particularly if digitalis toxicity is the cause).

6. These arrhythmias are usually quite resistant to treatment with standard class I or III agents.
7. Catheter ablation may be effective if a causative agent cannot be identified or treated.

V. The major ectopic arrhythmias

A. Wandering atrial pacemaker
  1. Mechanisms and causes
    a. Three or more ectopic pacemakers in the atria manifest themselves by default or usurpation.
    b. This arrhythmia is typically seen in young healthy persons, particularly athletes.
  2. Heart rate
    a. The atrial rate is 60–100.
    b. The ventricular response is regular.
  3. ECG morphology
    a. There are at least three P wave morphologies.
    b. There may be moderate variation in the atrial and ventricular rates.

Lead II—wandering atrial pacemaker

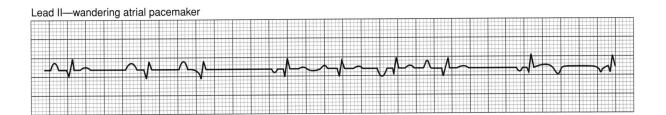

B. Ectopic atrial rhythms
  1. Mechanisms and causes
    a. A single ectopic atrial focus accelerates and usurps control from the sinus node.
    b. Digitalis toxicity, electrolyte abnormalities, ischemia, hypoxia, and chronic lung disease are typical causes.
  2. ECG morphology
    a. The P waves are of the same morphology but have an abnormal axis, indicating their ectopic origin.
    b. The atrial rate may be slightly irregular.
    c. AV block of varying degrees is frequently present (particularly if digitalis toxicity is the cause).
    d. Atrial tachycardia with AV block should be considered a manifestation of digitalis toxicity until proven otherwise.
    e. The atrial rate in atrial tachycardia is usually 140–200.
    f. Atrial tachycardia may be confused with atrial flutter, but the latter is usually faster and the baseline is not flat between the P waves.

Lead II—ectopic atrial bradycardia

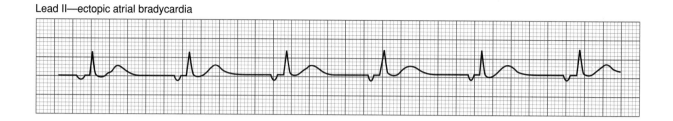

Lead II—atrial tachycardia with AV block and right bundle branch block. Note the rapid atrial rate with an abnormal P wave axis and the variable AV block. This patient's digoxin level was 3.7 mg/dL.

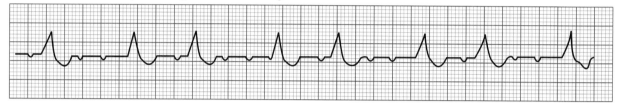

Lead II—atrial tachycardia with 3° AV block

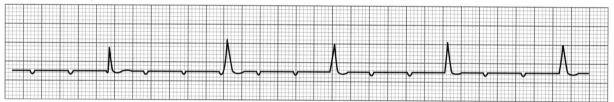

Lead V$_1$—atrial tachycardia with 3:1 AV block

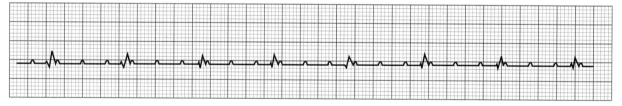

Lead II—atrial tachycardia

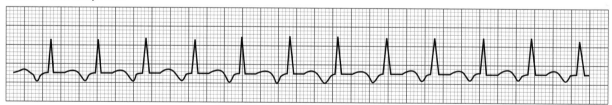

C. Multifocal atrial tachycardia
 1. Mechanisms and causes
  a. Caused by multiple ectopic atrial foci.
  b. Chronic lung disease, particularly when treated with theophylline, is usually the underlying clinical abnormality.
 2. ECG morphology
  a. There must be at least three P wave morphologies.
  b. The atrial rate may be quite irregular.
  c. The PR interval usually varies.
  d. The atrial rate must be greater than 100.
  e. There is typically 1:1 AV conduction.

Lead II—multifocal atrial tachycardia

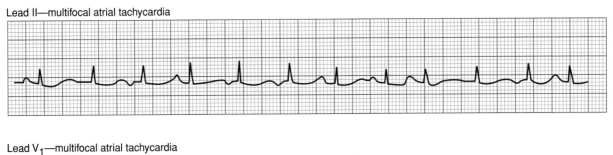

Lead V₁—multifocal atrial tachycardia

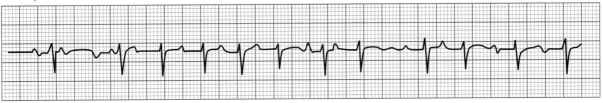

D. Ectopic junctional rhythms
 1. Mechanisms and causes
  a. A single focus in or near the AV node accelerates and usurps control from the sinus node.
  b. Digitalis toxicity, electrolyte abnormalities, ischemia, hypoxia, and chronic lung disease are typical causes.
 2. ECG morphology
  a. If P waves are visible, they demonstrate an abnormal axis and appear slightly before or after the QRS complex.
  b. Junctional tachycardia (rate > 60) (also known as accelerated junctional rhythm) should be considered a manifestation of digitalis toxicity until proven otherwise.
  c. Junctional tachycardia may be confused with atrial tachycardia, but the latter has a normal PR interval (>120 msec).

Lead II—accelerated junctional rhythm

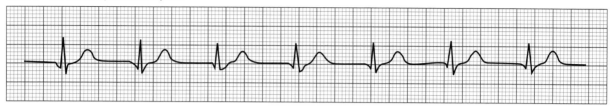

Lead II—sinus arrhythmia with a junctional escape mechanism

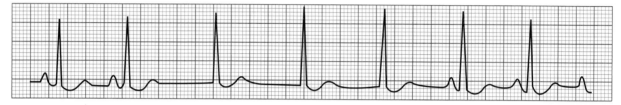

Lead II—junctional tachycardia versus PSVT

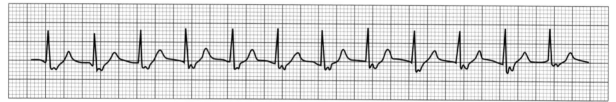

Lead V$_1$—atrial fibrillation with complete heart block and an accelerated junctional rhythm, highly suggestive of digitalis toxicity

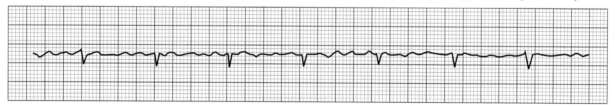

E. Ectopic ventricular rhythms
   1. Mechanisms and causes
      a. A single focus in the right or left ventricle, usually near the His-Purkinje fibers, accelerates and usurps control from the sinus node.
      b. Ischemia, electrolyte abnormalities, and dilated cardiomyopathies are typical causes.
      c. VT can also be associated with right ventricular dysplasia, a congenital condition affecting the right ventricular free wall and/or RV outflow tract (this abnormality may also produce reentrant VT).
   2. ECG morphology
      a. The ECG demonstrates a wide QRS tachycardia.
      b. There may be AV dissociation.
      c. In RV dysplasia, the ECG shows LBBB, right axis deviation, and T wave inversion over the right precordium.

Lead V_1—ectopic ventricular tachycardia in a 23-year-old woman, subsequently treated by radio frequency catheter ablation

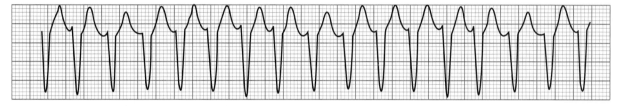

Summary of ectopic arrhythmias

ARRHYTHMIA	ECTOPIC RATE	ECG DESCRIPTION
Wandering Atrial Pacemaker	60–100	Multiple P wave morphologies (usually three or more), variable rate
Ectopic Atrial Rhythm	40–250	Regular P waves with abnormal axis, PR inverval > 120 msec, flat baseline between P waves, A:V conduction may be 1:1 or variable
Multifocal Atrial Tachycardia	100–180	At least 3 P wave morphologies, varying PR intervals, rate > 100
Junctional Rhythms	40–120	Regular ventricular rhythm with P waves slightly before, hidden inside, or after the QRS complex, PR interval < 120 msec
VT	120–250	Wide QRS tachycardia, regular ventricular rate

VI. Triggered activity

    A. Mechanisms of triggered activity
1. Triggered activity is initiated in conducting tissue by after-depolarizations.
2. Afterdepolarizations are oscillations of membrane voltage induced by one or more preceding action potentials.
3. If the afterdepolarization voltage reaches the membrane threshold potential, a sustained arrhythmia may result.
4. Patients with the congenital long QT syndromes or those treated with quinidine, procainamide, erythromycin, or some class III antiarrhythmic agents are at increased risk for triggered activity arrhythmias.
5. Triggered activity arrhythmias are exacerbated by hypokalemia or hypomagnesemia.

    B. Properties of triggered activity arrhythmias
1. Sustained, rapid ventricular tachycardia may be caused by triggered activity.
2. Another form of VT, torsade de pointes, also called polymorphic ventricular tachycardia, is characterized by a rapid, irregular ventricular rate and a cyclically changing morphology.
3. The treatment of these arrhythmias usually involves treatment of the underlying cardiac disease, correction of an electrolyte abnormality, or cessation of an offending drug.
4. Some of these arrhythmias respond to verapamil, ventricular pacing, or alpha adrenergic blockade.

Lead V$_5$—sinus rhythm with frequent salvos of rapid ventricular tachycardia which degenerates in the second strip to torsade de pointes

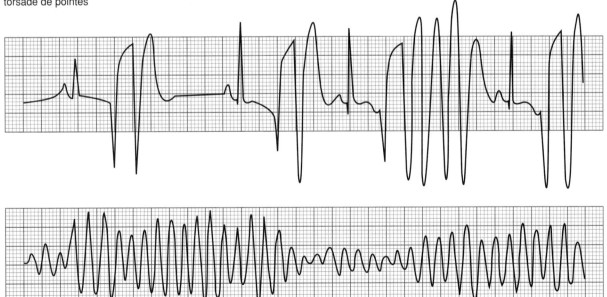

Day 6 ECG 1

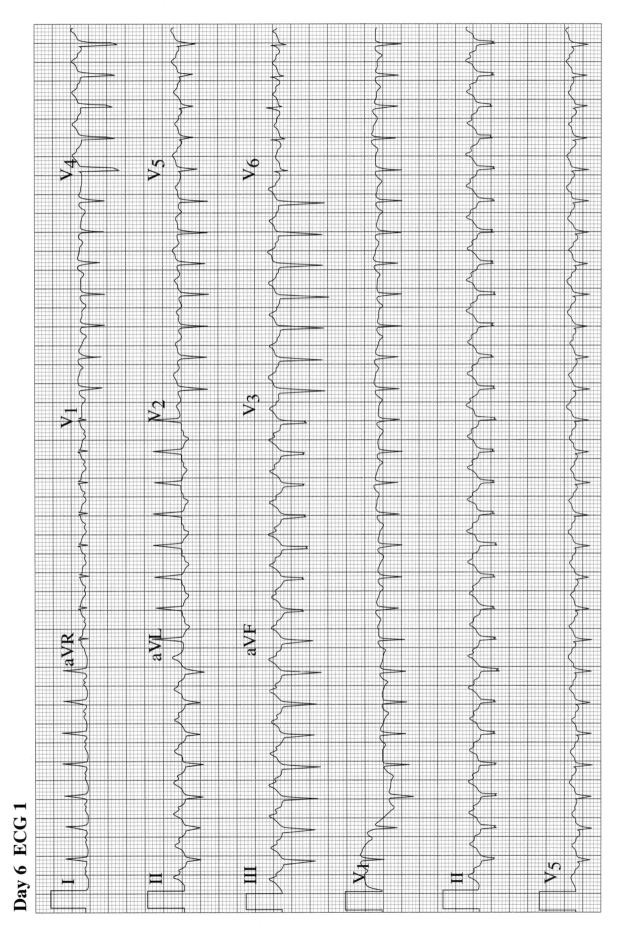

Day 6 ECG 2

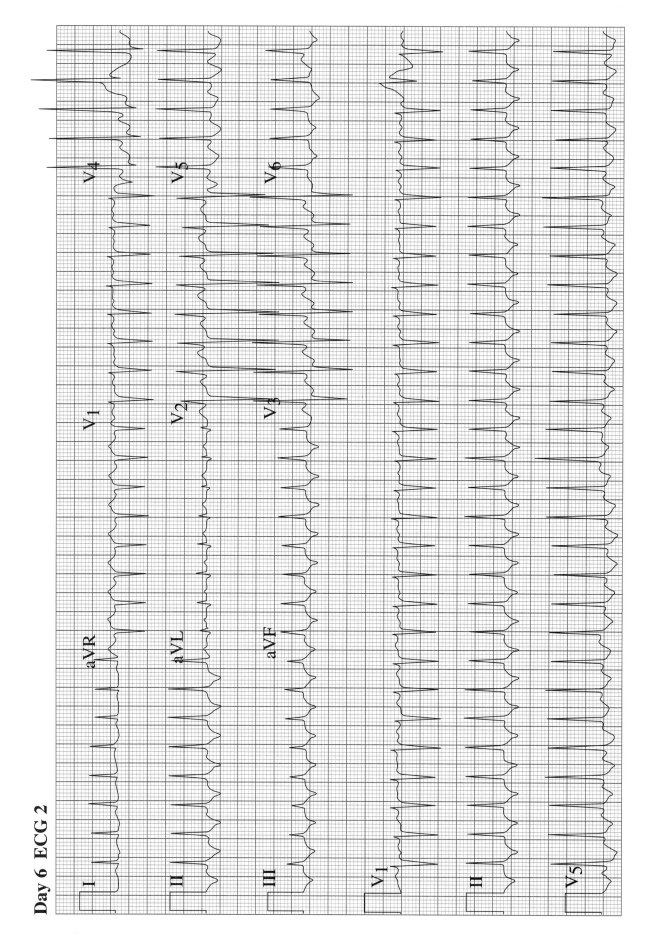

Day 6 ECG 3

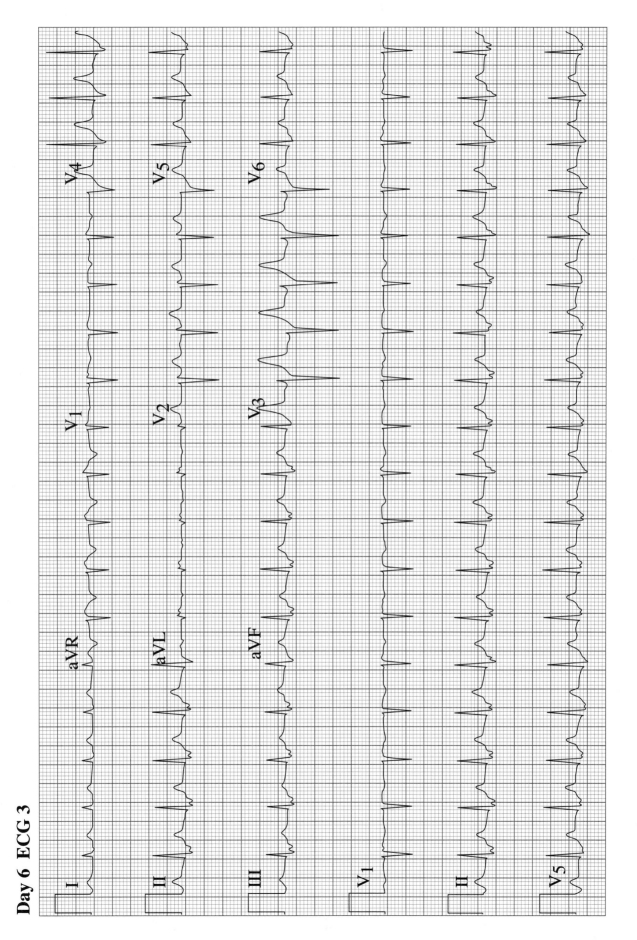

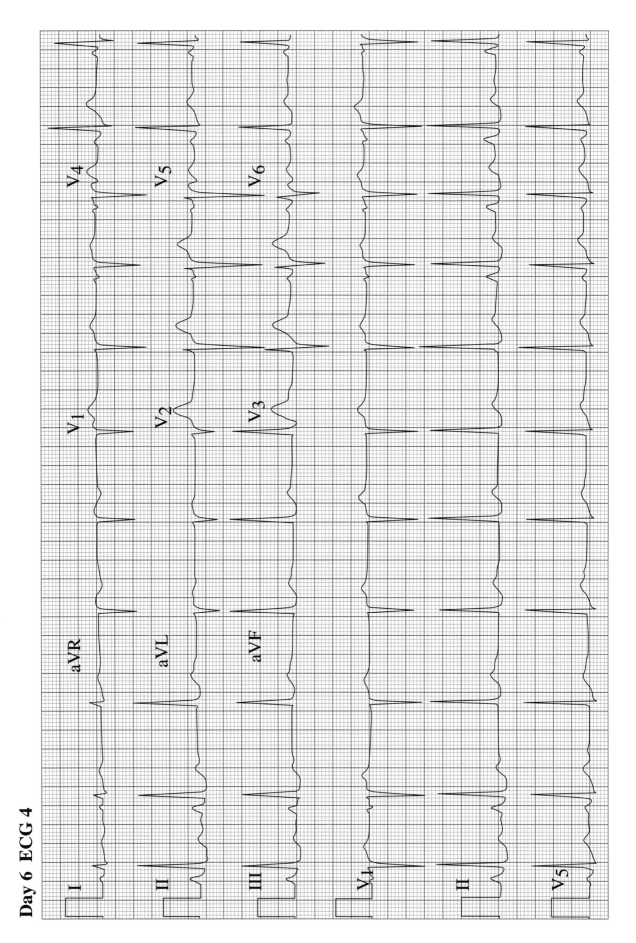

Day 6 ECG 4

132

Day 6 ECG 5

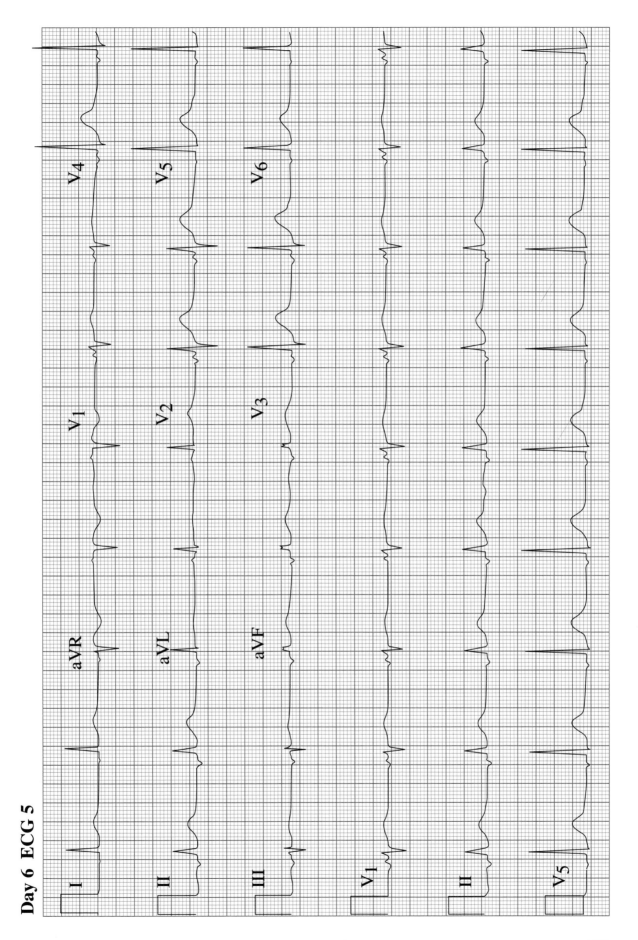

Day 6 ECG 6

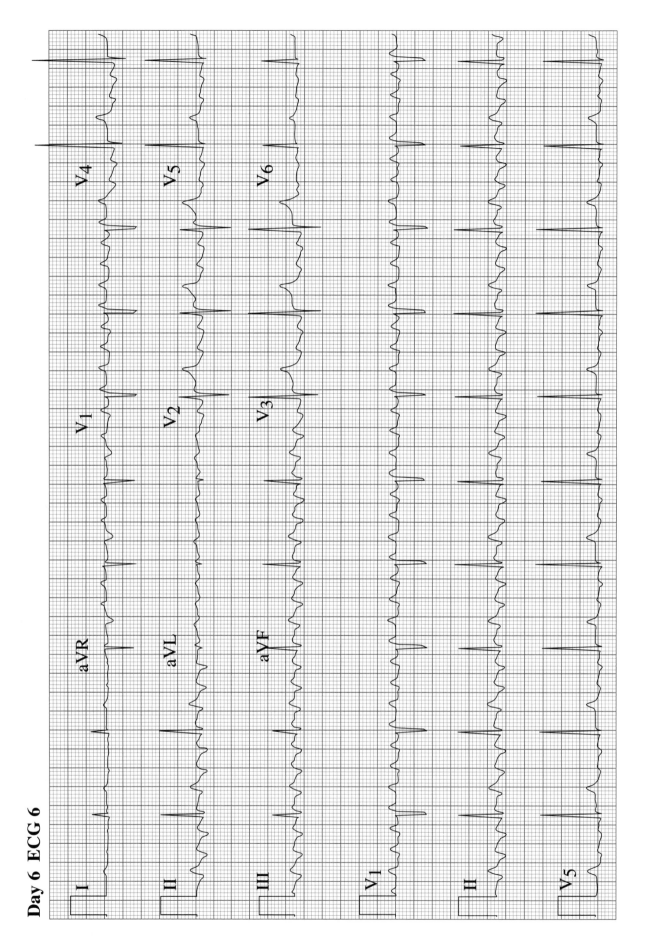

Day 6 ECG 7

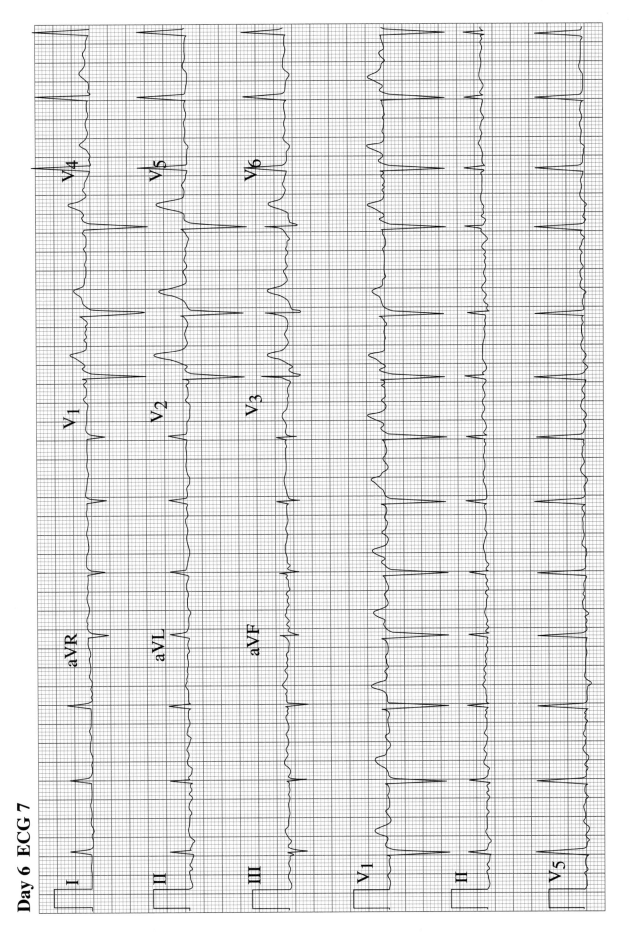

Day 6 ECG 8

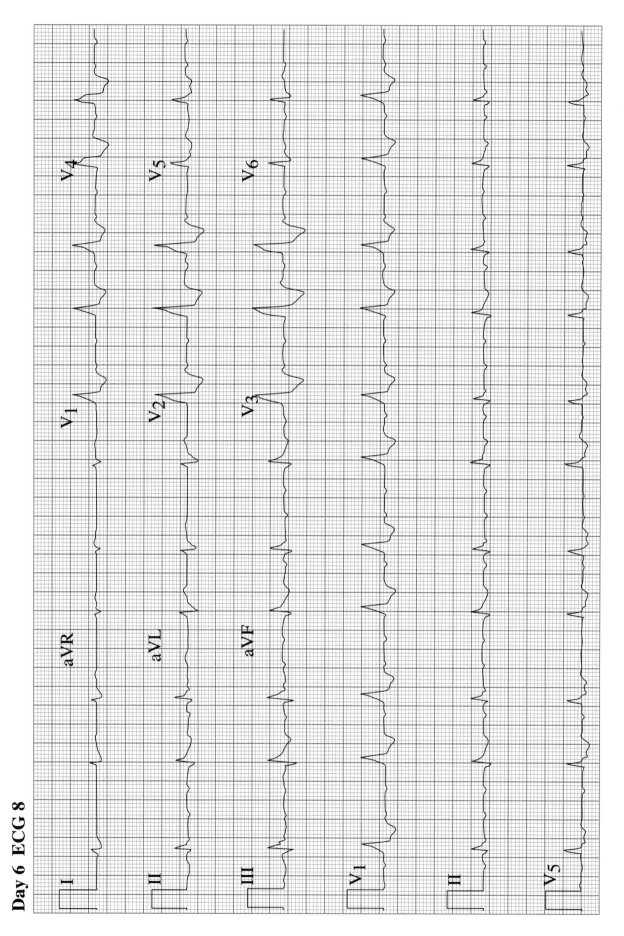

Day 6 ECG 9

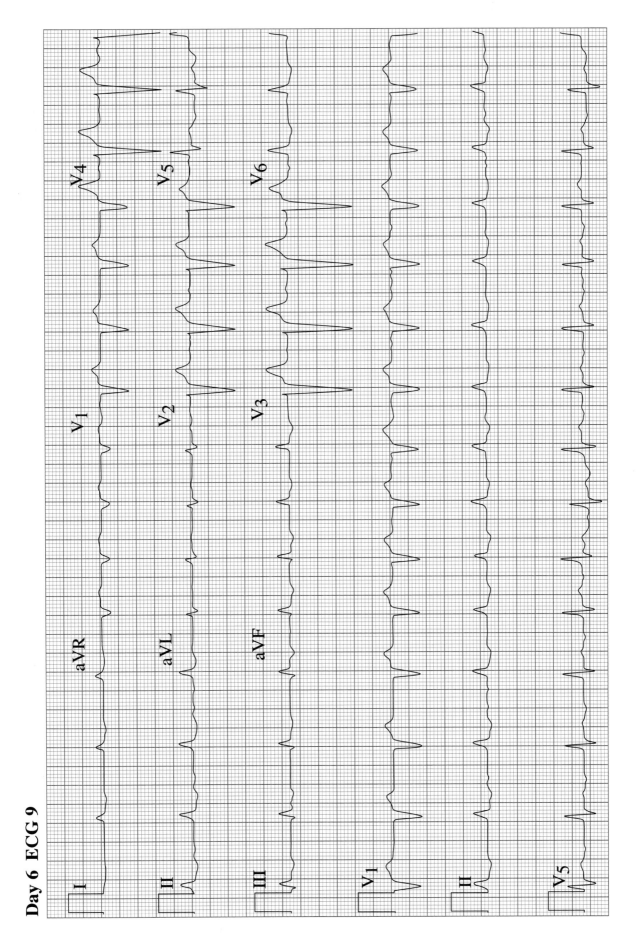

Day 6 ECG 10

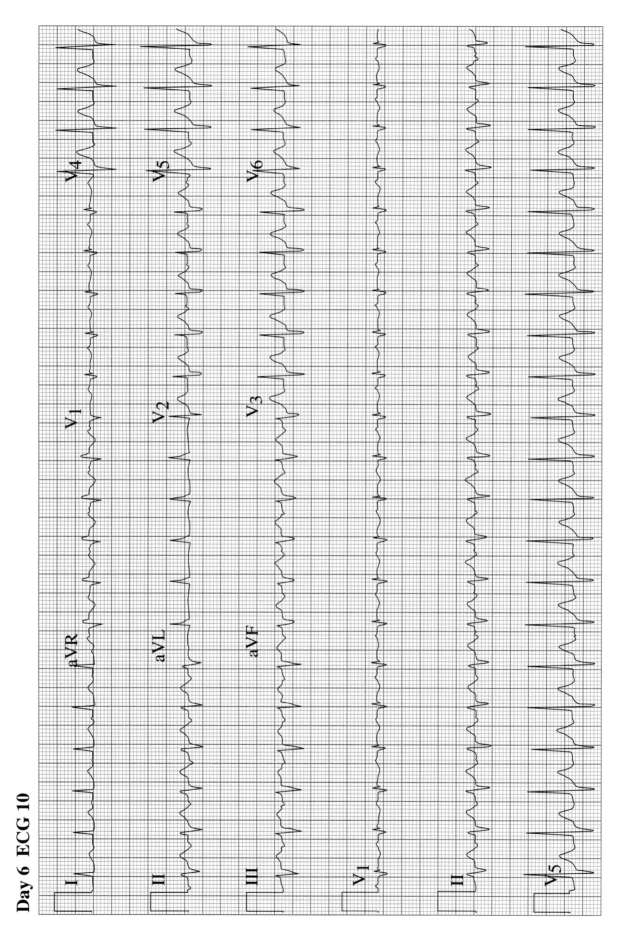

138

Day 6 ECG 11

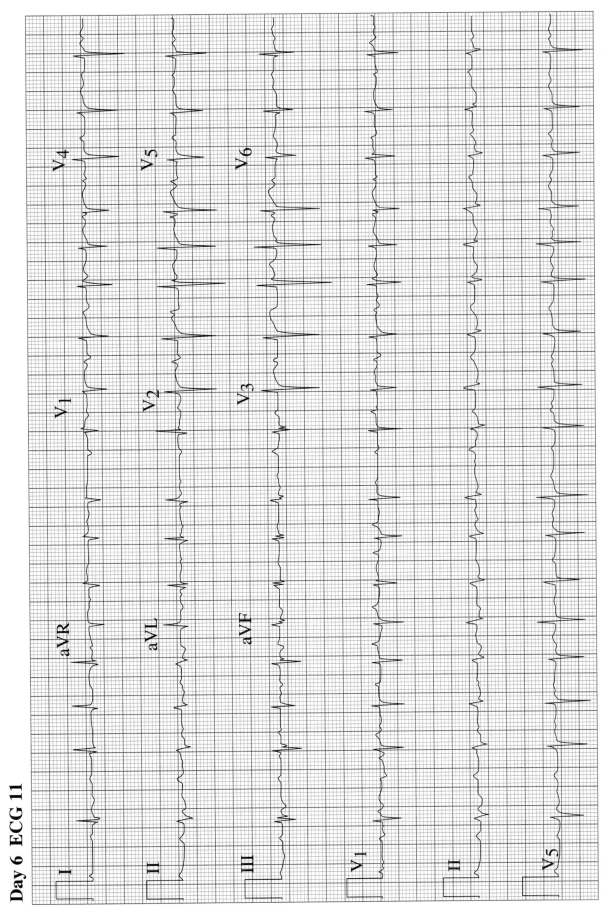

Day 6 ECG 12

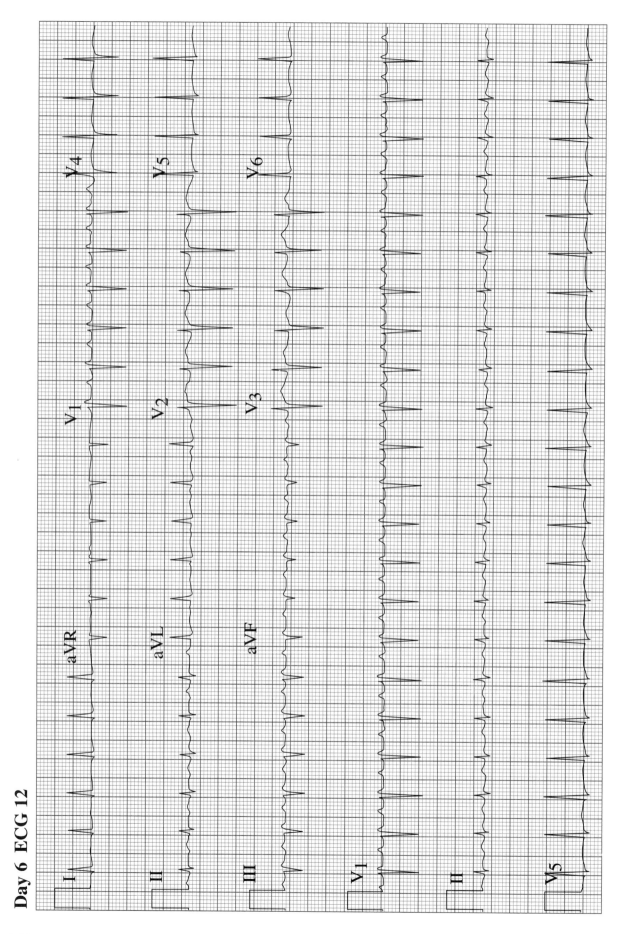

Day 6 ECG 13

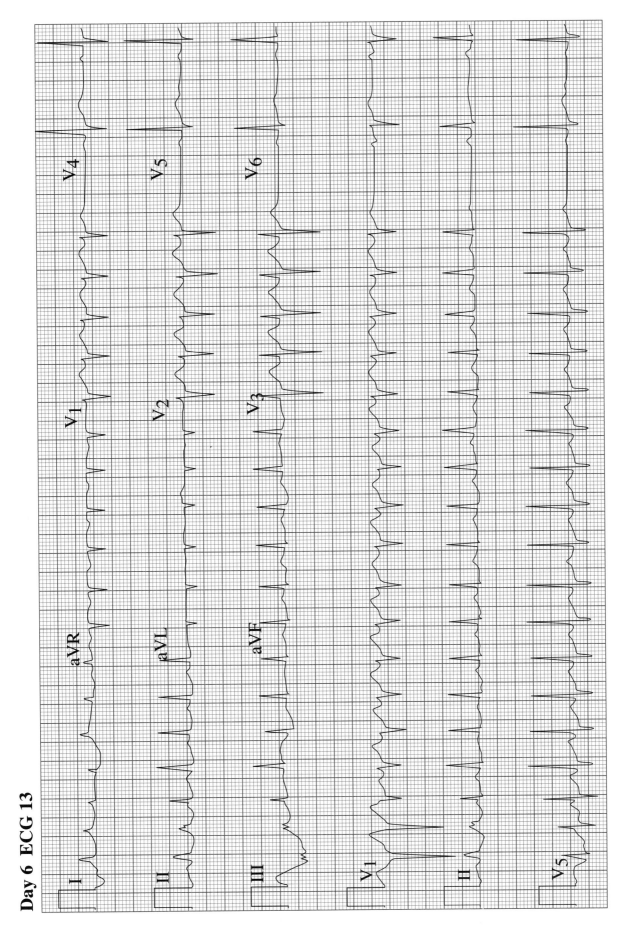

Day 6 ECG 14

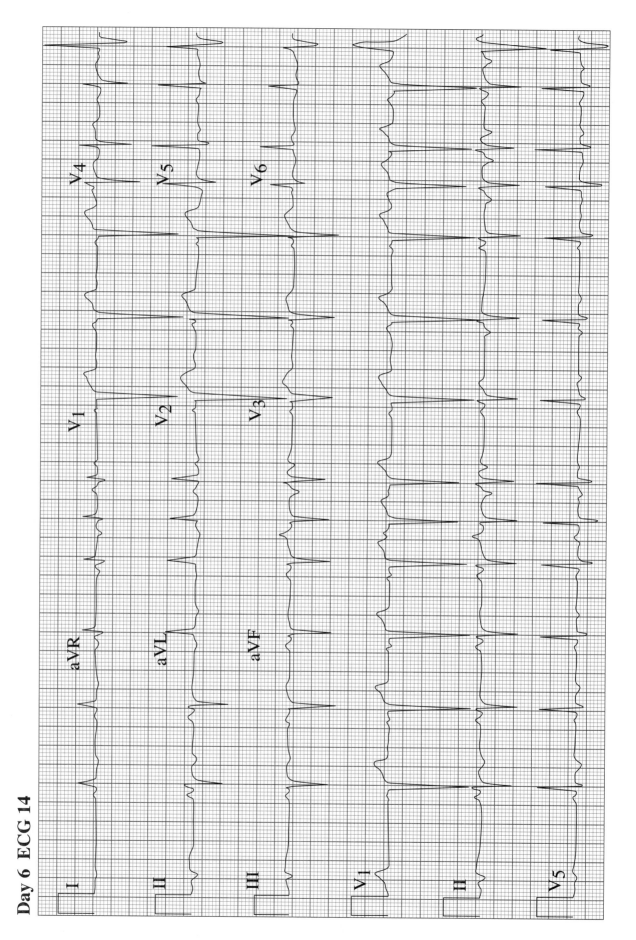

I   aVR   V1   V4

II   aVL   V2   V5

III   aVF   V3   V6

V1

II

V5

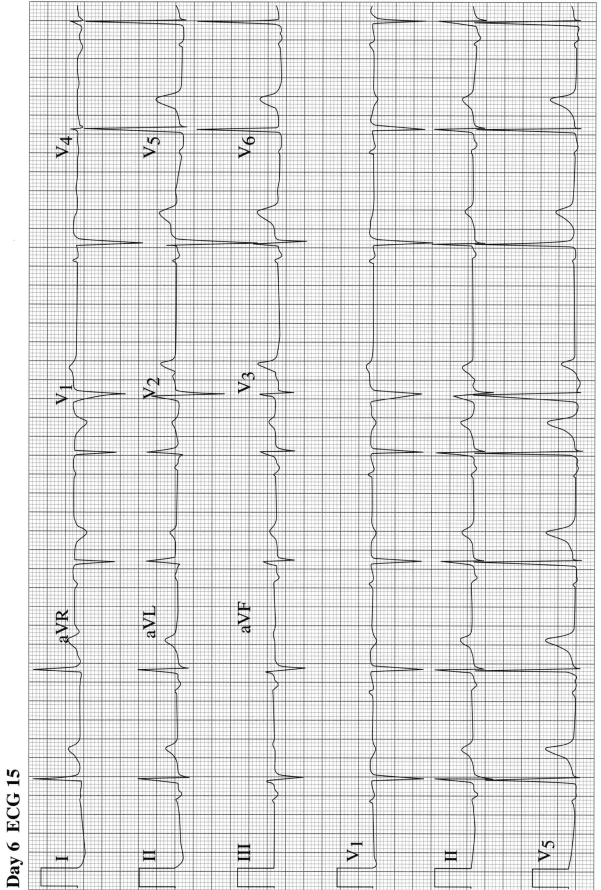

Day 6 ECG 16

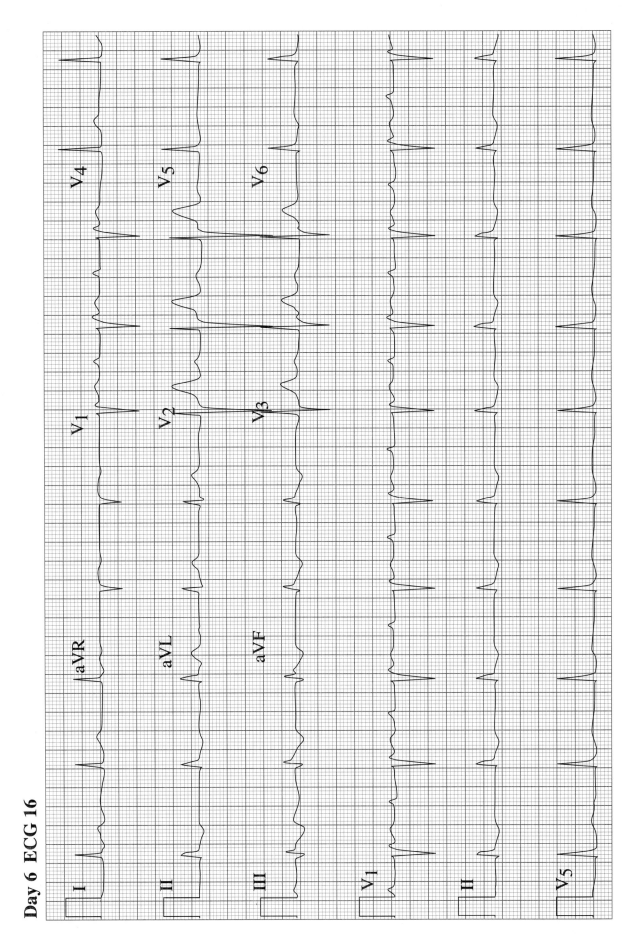

Day 6 ECG 17

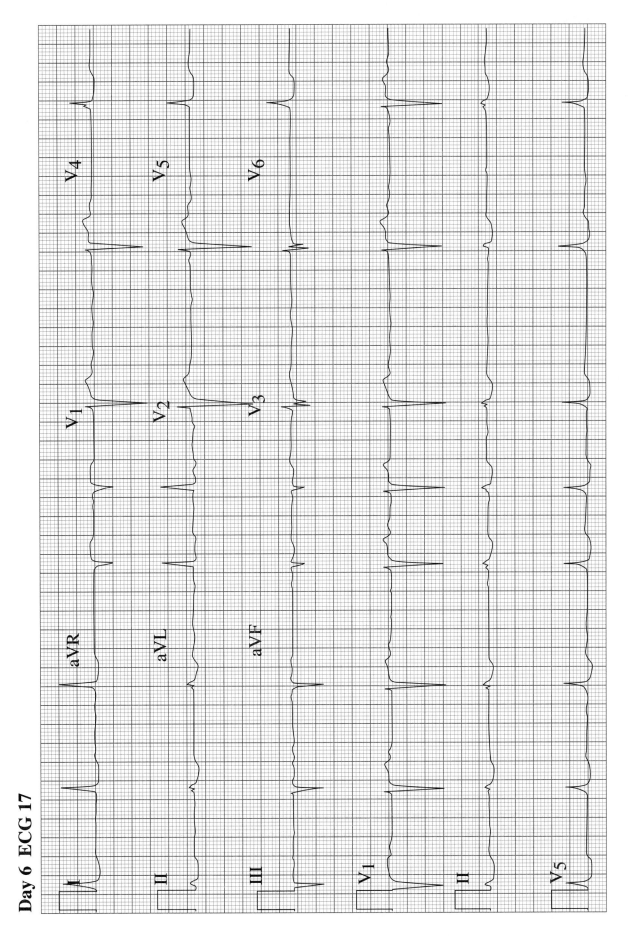

Day 6 ECG 18

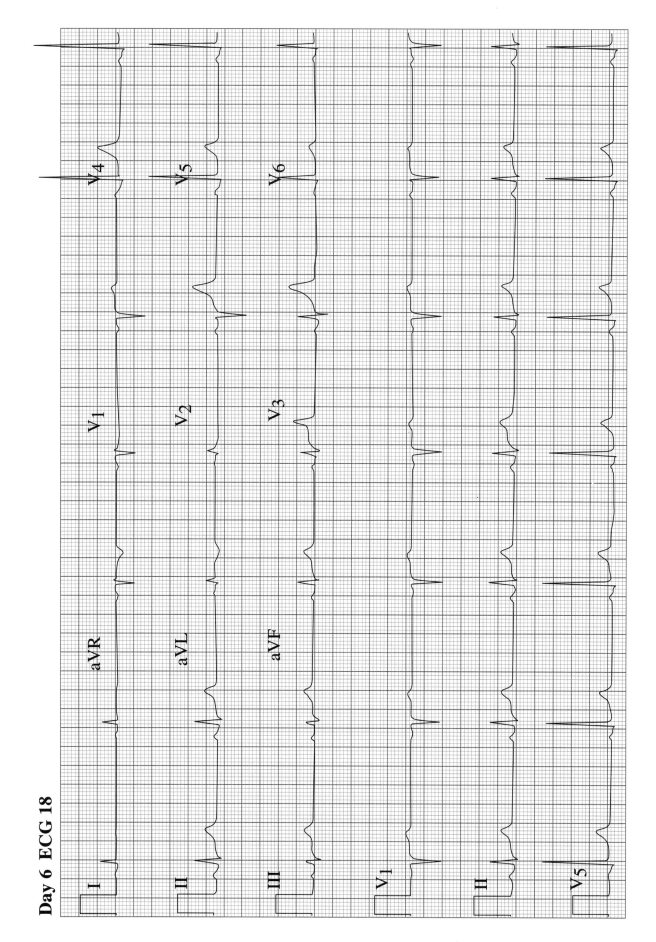

Day 6 ECG 19

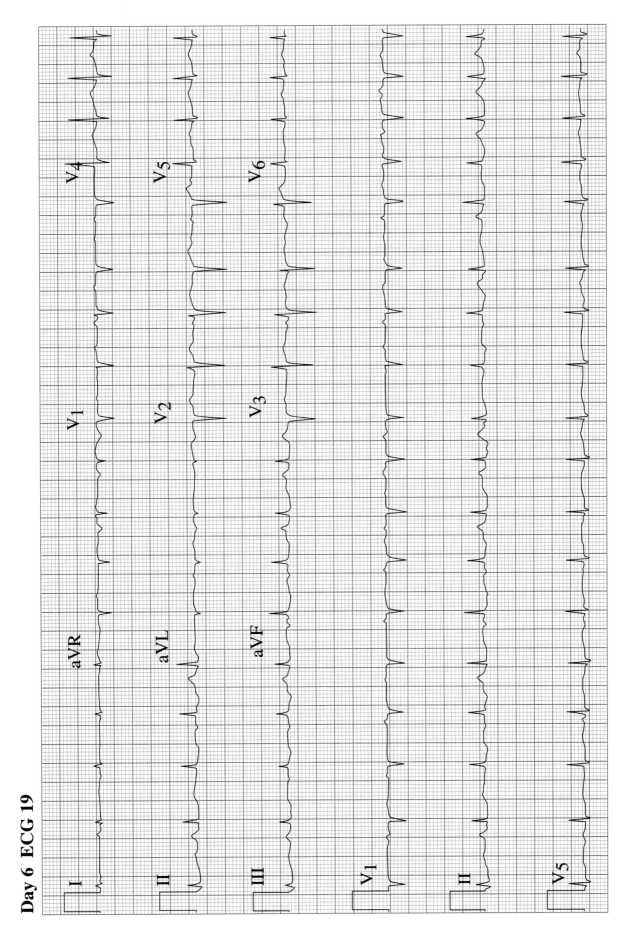

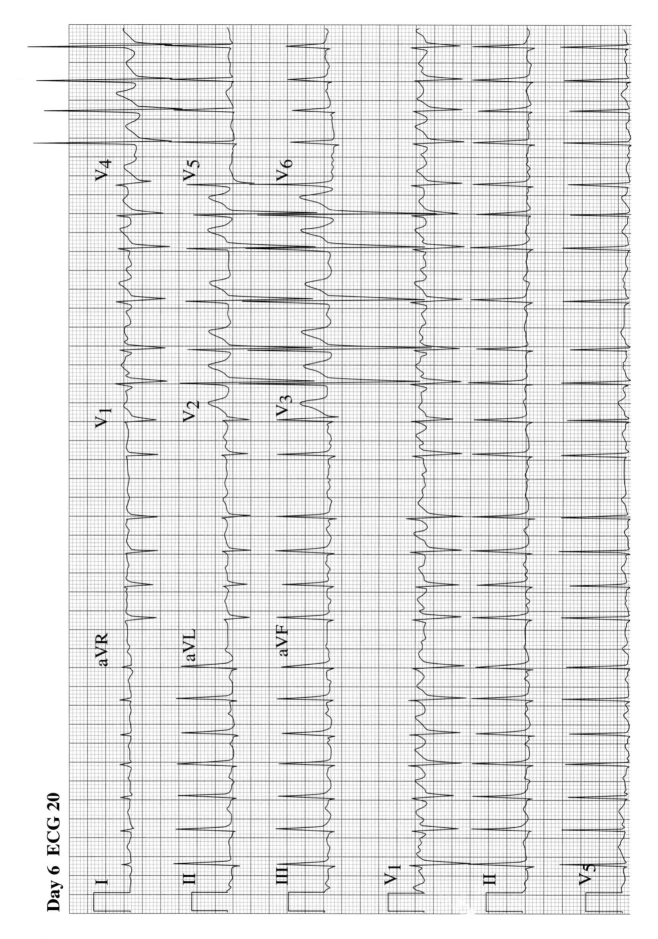

Day 6 ECG 20

148

Day 6 ECG 21

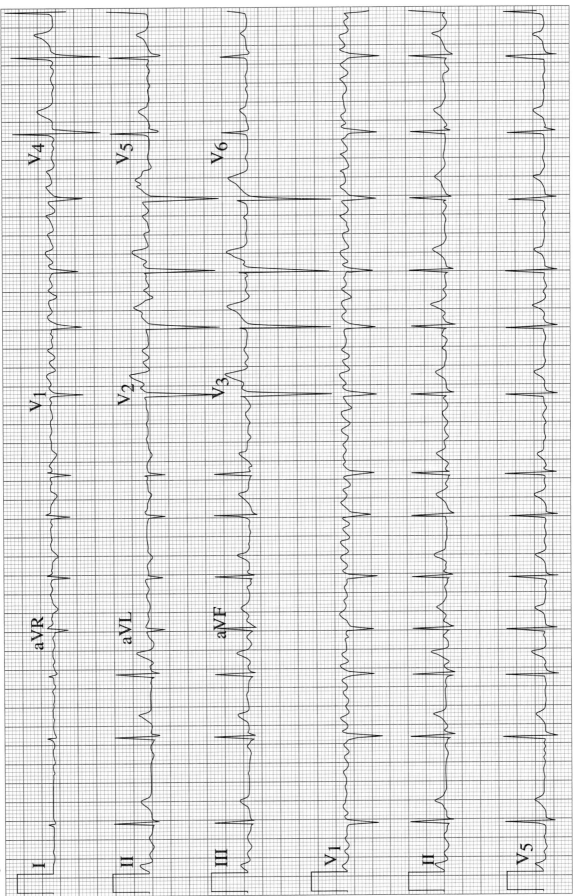

Day 6 ECG 22

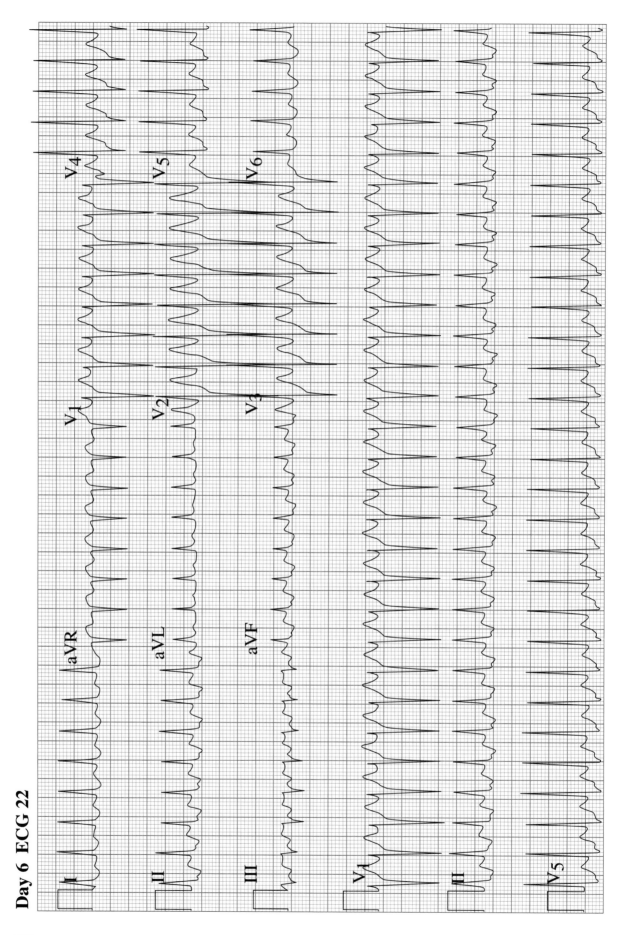

Day 6 ECG 23

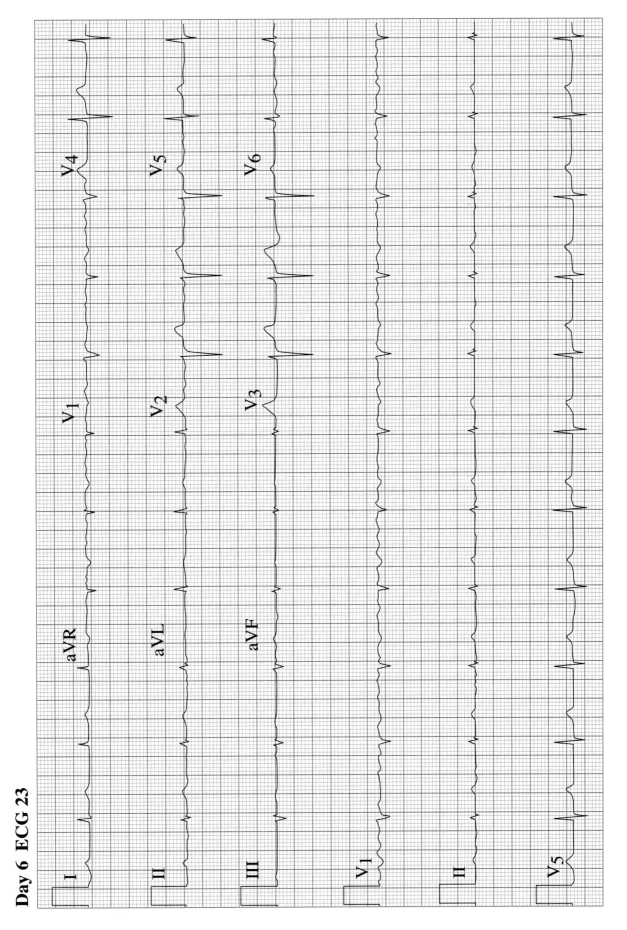

Day 6 ECG 24

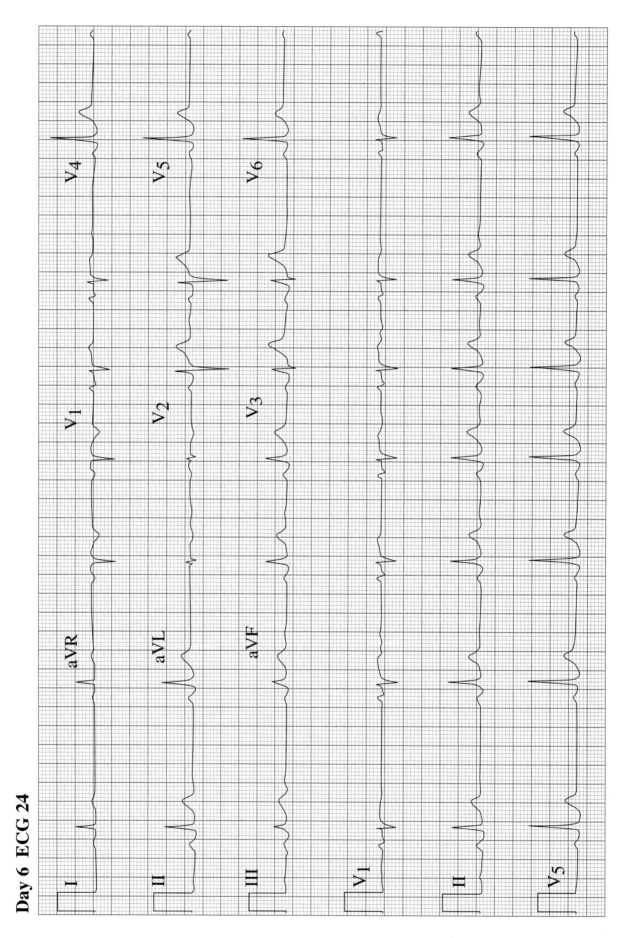

Day 6 ECG 25

** Chest leads are at half standard**

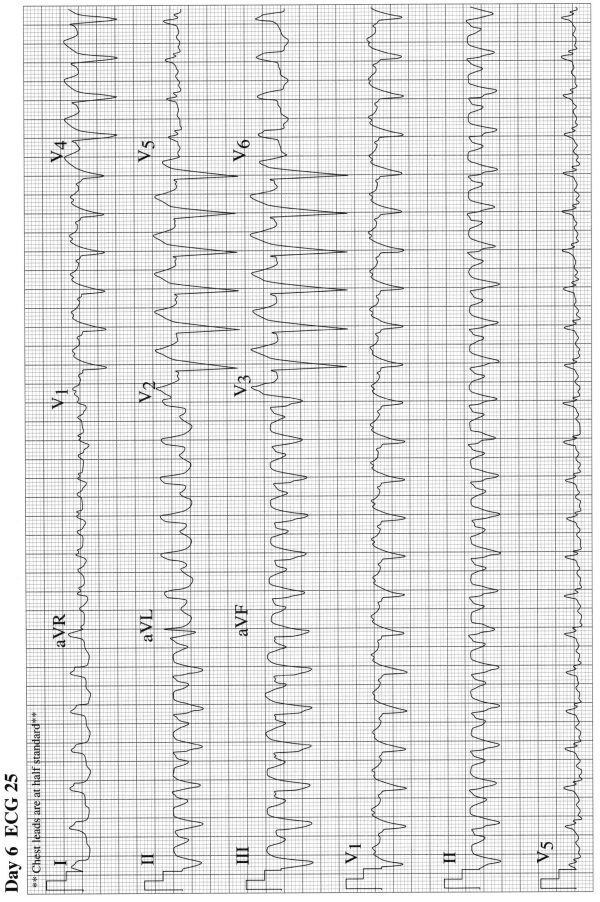

I aVR V1 V4

II aVL V2 V5

III aVF V3 V6

V1

II

V5

Day 6 ECG 26

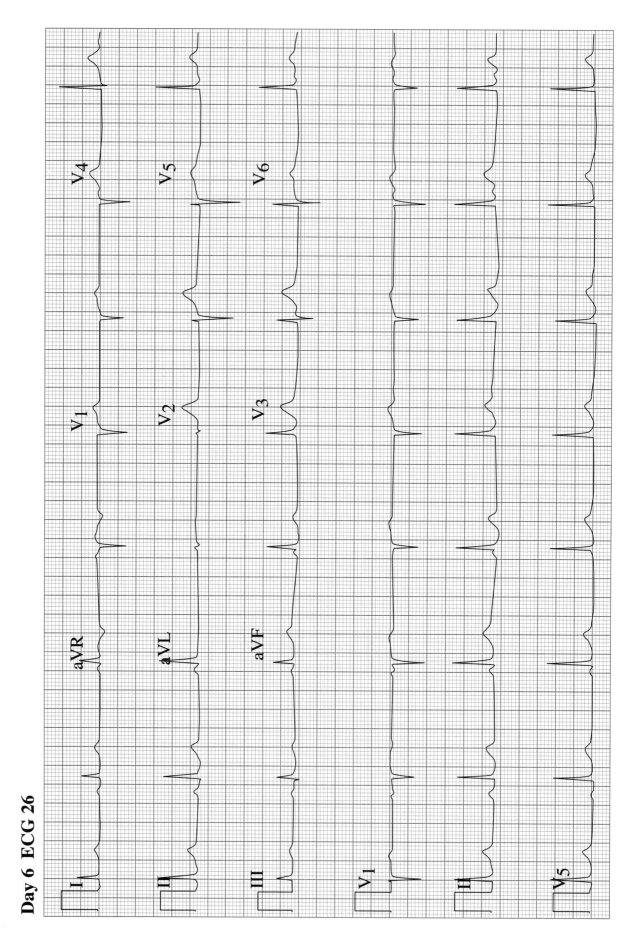

Day 6 ECG 27

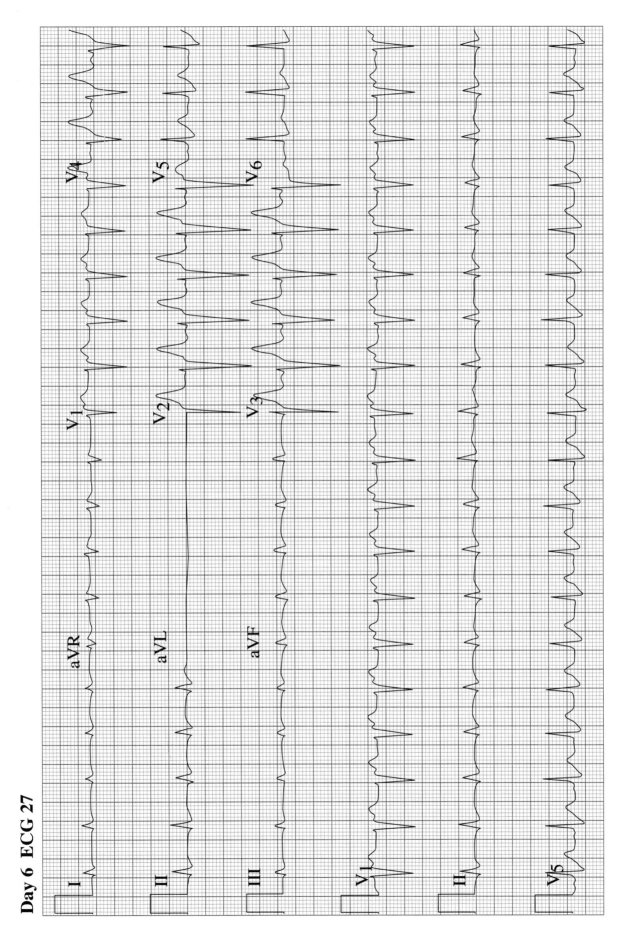

Day 6 ECG 28

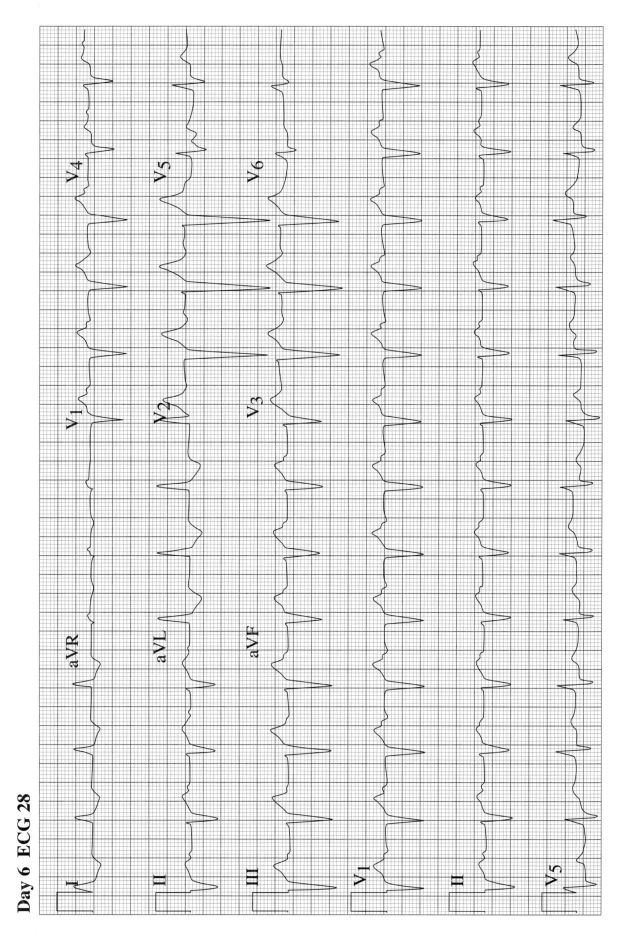

Day 6 ECG 29

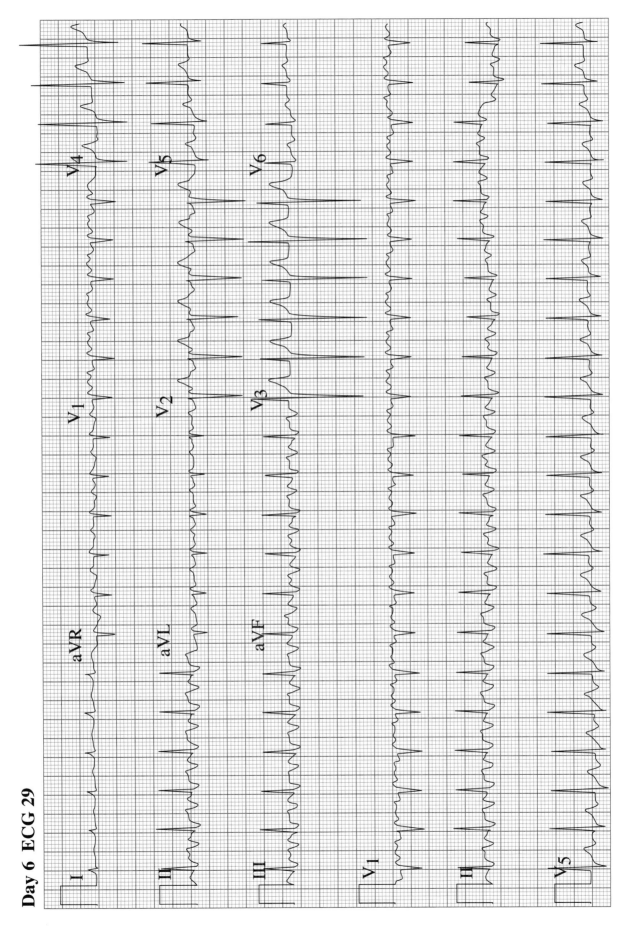

Day 6 ECG 30

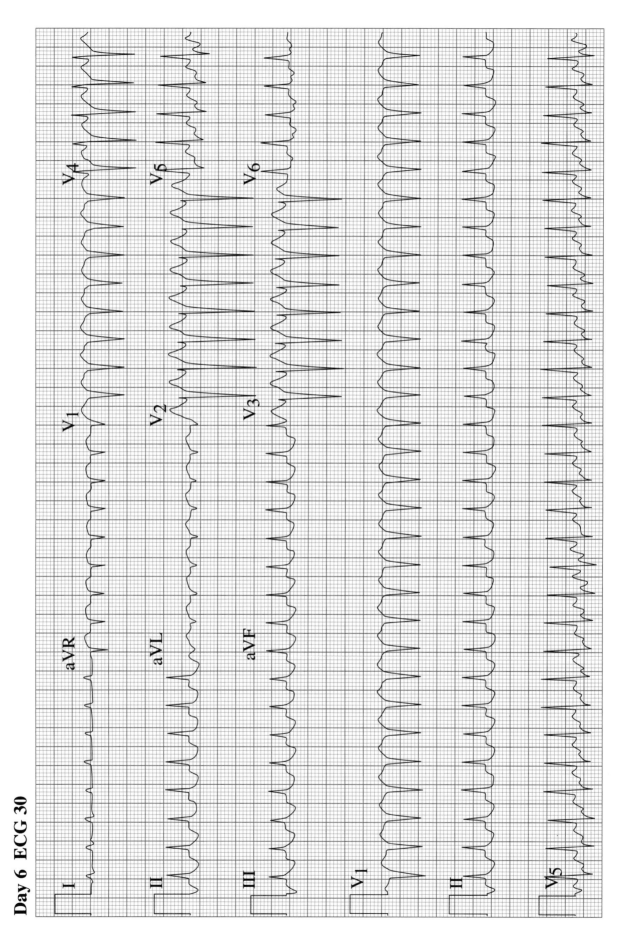

I aVR V1 V4

II aVL V2 V5

III aVF V3 V6

V1

II

V5

Day 6
ECG Interpretations and Discussion

Day 6 ECG 1
   Sinus tachycardia
   Left axis deviation
   Inferior MI, age undetermined
   Anterior MI, age undetermined

Even though the rate is very fast (about 170), there are P waves with a normal axis preceding each QRS complex. It is unusual for sinus tachycardia to have this rate unless the patient has just finished exercising or is very ill. There are Q waves in the inferior and anterior leads consistent with previous infarctions in those locations.

Day 6 ECG 2
   PSVT

There are inverted P waves between the QRS complexes. The distance of the P waves from the QRS complex strongly supports the uncommon form of PSVT, in which there is antegrade conduction down the fast pathway of the AV node and retrograde conduction up the slow pathway.

Day 6 ECG 3
   PSVT

There are inverted P waves immediately following the QRS complexes. The short distance of the P waves from the QRS complex strongly supports the common form of PSVT, in which there is antegrade conduction down the slow pathway of the AV node and retrograde conduction up the fast pathway.

Day 6 ECG 4
   Sinus rhythm with sinus arrhythmia and a junctional escape mechanism
   Right atrial abnormality
   Nonspecific ST and T wave changes

There is underlying sinus rhythm but the sinus mechanism slows after the first two beats and a junctional escape rhythm takes over. This lasts until the last four beats when the sinus mechanism speeds up and reasserts control. The reason for the sinus slowing is not apparent. There are tall pointed P waves in II and III, consistent with right atrial abnormality. There is some sagging of the ST segments in several leads.

Day 6 ECG 5
   Ectopic atrial bradycardia
   Nonspecific ST changes

The P waves have an unusual axis (inverted in II and aVF), and the PR interval is greater than 120 msec, consistent with an ectopic atrial rhythm. The rate is less than 60.

Day 6 ECG 6
Atrial flutter with 4:1 AV conduction

There are typical sawtooth flutter waves in multiple leads.

Day 6 ECG 7
Atrial fibrillation
Nonspecific ST and T wave changes

There is an irregular baseline and an irregular ventricular response.

Day 6 ECG 8
Atrial tachycardia with variable AV block
Right bundle branch block
Inferior MI, age undetermined

The atrial rate is about 170 and the P waves have an unusual axis. There is variable AV conduction. The QRS complexes have a right bundle branch block morphology. There are Q waves in the inferior leads consistent with a previous inferior MI. This arrhythmia has a 50% specificity for digitalis toxicity.

Day 6 ECG 9
Atrial fibrillation
Nonspecific intraventricular conduction defect

There is an irregular ventricular rhythm and no obvious P waves, consistent with atrial fibrillation. The QRS duration is greater than 120 msec, but the QRS complexes do not fit the definitions of right or left bundle branch block.

Day 6 ECG 10
PSVT
Left axis deviation

There are inverted P waves between the QRS complexes. The distance of the P waves from the QRS complex strongly supports the uncommon form of PSVT, in which there is antegrade conduction down the fast pathway of the AV node and retrograde conduction up the slow pathway. The QRS complex is upright in I, but downward in aVF and II, indicating left axis deviation.

Day 6 ECG 11
Multifocal atrial tachycardia
Nonspecific ST and T wave changes

There are at least three P wave morphologies, varying PR interval, and a ventricular rate greater than 100, indicating multifocal atrial tachycardia.

Day 6 ECG 12
  Atrial flutter with 2:1 AV block

This regular supraventricular (as indicated by the narrow QRS complexes) tachycardia has a rate of 150. This strongly implies atrial flutter with 2:1 AV conduction. The atrial rate of nearly 300 can be discerned in V_1.

Day 6 ECG 13
  PSVT with subsequent return to sinus rhythm

PSVT is present during the first part of the ECG. It terminates suddenly and is replaced by sinus rhythm. The paroxysmal nature of reentrant arrhythmias is well demonstrated in this ECG.

Day 6 ECG 14
  Wandering atrial pacemaker
  Ventricular extrasystoles
  Left axis deviation
  Left ventricular hypertrophy with repolarization abnormalities

There are several P wave morphologies indicating wandering atrial pacemaker. There is a wide QRS beat consistent with a ventricular extrasystole. The QRS is upright in I and downward in aVF and II, indicating left axis deviation. There are voltage criteria for left ventricular hypertrophy and ST segment and T wave repolarization abnormalities.

Day 6 ECG 15
  Ectopic atrial bradycardia
  Ventricular extrasystoles
  Left ventricular hypertrophy

The P waves have an unusual axis (inverted in II and aVF), and the PR interval is greater than 120 msec, consistent with an ectopic atrial rhythm. The rate is less than 60. There is a wide QRS beat consistent with a ventricular extrasystole. There are voltage criteria for left ventricular hypertrophy.

Day 6 ECG 16
  Atrial tachycardia with 2:1 AV block
  Inferior MI, age undetermined

There is atrial tachycardia at a rate of about 120, best seen in V_1. The P wave axis is abnormal. There are Q waves in III and aVF suggesting a previous inferior MI.

Day 6 ECG 17
   Atrial fibrillation with slow ventricular response
   Inferior MI, age undetermined
   Nonspecific ST and T wave changes

There is an irregular baseline and a very slow irregular ventricular response, consistent with atrial fibrillation. There are Q waves in III and aVF indicating a previous inferior MI. There is diffuse ST segment sagging, suggesting digitalis effect.

Day 6 ECG 18
   Sinus bradycardia

Day 6 ECG 19
   Multifocal atrial tachycardia
   Low voltage in the limb leads
   Nonspecific ST changes

There are at least three P wave morphologies, varying PR interval, and a ventricular rate greater than 100, indicating multifocal atrial tachycardia. The absolute value of the QRS complexes in the limb leads is less than 5 mm.

Day 6 ECG 20
   Atrial fibrillation with rapid ventricular response
   Nonspecific T wave abnormalities

There is a rapid irregular rhythm. During somewhat longer intervals, the irregular baseline can be appreciated.

Day 6 ECG 21
   Atrial fibrillation
   Nonspecific ST and T wave changes

There is an irregular baseline and an irregular ventricular response.

Day 6 ECG 22
   PSVT
   Left ventricular hypertrophy
   Marked ST segment and T wave changes suggesting ischemia

There is a rapid regular rhythm. Inverted P waves can be identified in II, suggesting the common form of PSVT. There are voltage criteria for left ventricular hypertrophy. There is marked ST segment depression in several leads which may be due to left ventricular hypertrophy, but is strongly suggestive of ischemia.

Day 6 ECG 23
  Atrial fibrillation
  Accelerated junctional rhythm
  Low voltage in the limb leads

There is an irregular baseline without obvious P waves indicating atrial fibrillation. There is a regular narrow ventricular rhythm at a rate of 72. This suggests that there is complete heart block and an independent accelerated junctional rhythm. This situation is strongly suggestive of digitalis toxicity, which accounts for the heart block and the accelerated junctional rhythm. The absolute value of the QRS complexes in the limb leads is less than 5 mm.

Day 6 ECG 24
  Sinus rhythm with marked sinus arrhythmia
  Nonspecific ST and T wave changes

There is more than a 10% variation in the intervals between beats, indicating sinus arrhythmia. This condition is usually associated with an exaggerated respiratory variation.

Day 6 ECG 25
  Atrial flutter with 2:1 AV block
  Left bundle branch block

This is a wide QRS tachycardia, but regular P waves at a rate of about 280 can be seen in V_1, indicating atrial flutter with 2:1 AV block. The QRS complex is greater than 120 msec and fulfills criteria for left bundle branch block. Note that the chest leads are at half standard.

Day 6 ECG 26
  Severe sinus bradycardia with a competing junctional rhythm

There is a very slow sinus rhythm and a slightly faster competing junctional rhythm. There is AV dissociation, but not third degree AV block.

Day 6 ECG 27
  PSVT
  Nonspecific intraventricular conduction defect

There are P waves following the QRS complexes in V_1, suggesting PSVT. This arrhythmia could also be accelerated junctional rhythm, but the rate is quite fast and PSVT is far more common. Vagal maneuvers or intravenous adenosine could be very useful in determining the rhythm.

Day 6 ECG 28
   Sinus rhythm with very long first degree AV block
   Left axis deviation
   Nonspecific intraventricular conduction defect

The PR interval is much greater than 200 msec, indicating first degree AV block. It is important to recognize that the P waves represent sinus rhythm (note the normal P wave axis), and not retrograde atrial activation from junctional rhythm.

Day 6 ECG 29
   Atrial flutter with 2:1 AV block

There are obvious sawtooth flutter waves in the inferior leads and V_1.

Day 6 ECG 30
   PSVT
   Nonspecific ST and T wave changes

This is a regular very rapid narrow complex rhythm. No P waves are apparent. The rate of 200 strongly suggests PSVT. Vagal maneuvers or intravenous adenosine would be very useful.

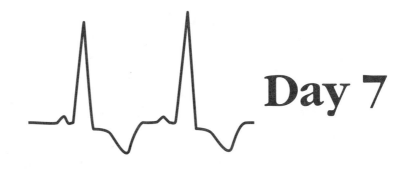

Day 7

Extrasystoles and Preexcitation Syndromes

I. Extrasystoles

   A. Mechanisms of extrasystoles
      1. Reentry
         a. Most extrasystoles, particularly if they are monomorphic, bear a constant relationship to the preceding QRS complex (a fixed coupling interval).
         b. The vast majority of these complexes represent a reentrant mechanism (each beat represents one trip around a reentrant pathway).
      2. Parasystole
         a. Parasystole occurs when an ectopic focus fires independently of the basic rhythm.
         b. If the basic rhythm is not reset by the ectopic focus, the focus is said to be protected (ie, electrical information can get out of the focus but it is not affected by the wave of normal depolarization going by).
         c. There is a constant interval between ectopic depolarizations, but the ectopic focus will manifest itself only when it finds the atrium or ventricle not refractory.
         d. Parasystole is very uncommon.
      3. Escape
         a. Escape is a normal phenomenon which occurs when there is a sufficient pause to allow a lower pacemaker to depolarize.
         b. Common examples are junctional or ventricular escape mechanisms.
      4. Unclassified—some extrasystoles do not fall easily into any of these categories and may remain undiagnosed.

   B. Atrial extrasystoles
      1. Most atrial extrasystoles are reentrant.
      2. Atrial extrasystoles are preceded by a P wave which may have normal or abnormal morphology.
      3. The QRS complex is narrow unless there is a preexisting intraventricular conduction defect.
      4. Occasionally, the QRS complex may be wide (aberrant) when one of the bundle branches is not fully repolarized.

5. An atrial extrasystole usually resets the sinus mechanism and therefore is not followed by a compensatory pause (see below).
6. If an atrial extrasystole is very early, the ventricle may be refractory and not depolarize ("the commonest cause of a pause is a nonconducted atrial extrasystole"—Marriott, from Wagner G. *Marriott's Practical Electrocardiography*. 9th ed. Baltimore: Williams & Wilkins; 1994:234).

Lead II—normal sinus rhythm with an isolated atrial extrasystole

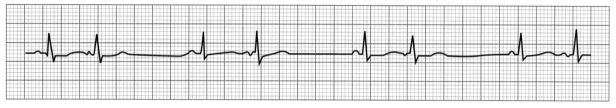

Lead II—normal sinus rhythm with atrial bigeminy. Note that the P waves preceding the extrasystolic beats are abnormal.

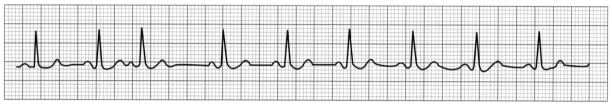

Lead II—normal sinus rhythm with regular atrial extrasystoles. The arrows indicate an additional nonconducted P wave superimposed on the top of the T waves.

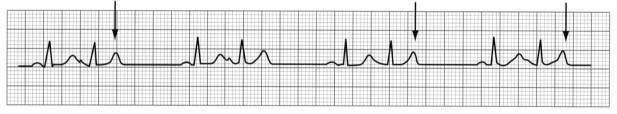

Lead II—normal sinus rhythm with a single aberrantly conducted atrial extrasystole. Note the P wave preceding the wide QRS complex.

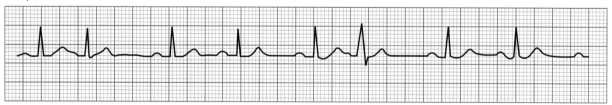

Lead II—sinus rhythm with two nonconducted atrial extrasystoles (first two arrows). The last arrow indicates a junctional escape beat after the long interval.

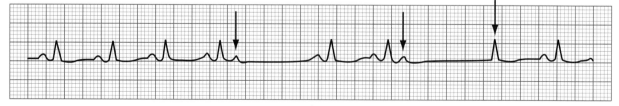

C. Ventricular extrasystoles
   1. Most ventricular extrasystoles are also reentrant.
   2. Ventricular extrasystoles are not preceded by a P wave.
   3. The QRS complex is obviously wide.
   4. Ventricular extrasystoles usually do not reset the atrial rate and are frequently followed by a compensatory pause.
   5. A ventricular extrasystole may cause retrograde depolarization of the AV node, which results in a lengthening of the subsequent PR interval—a phenomenon known as concealed retrograde conduction.

Lead V$_1$—normal sinus rhythm with a single ventricular extrasystole. The interval between the normal complexes surrounding the extrasystole (2x) is twice the interval between the normal complexes (x). This demonstrates the typical *compensatory pause* associated with ventricular extrasystoles.

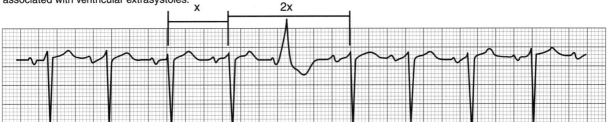

Lead II—normal sinus rhythm with a single ventricular extrasystole. The interval between the normal complexes surrounding the extrasystole is less than twice the interval between other complexes (x). A retrograde P wave (arrow) from the extrasystole has reset the sinus mechanism so there is *not* a compensatory pause.

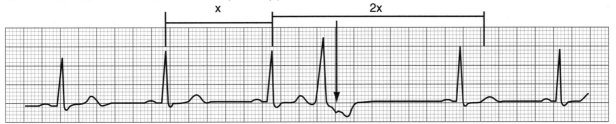

Lead II—normal sinus rhythm with a single ventricular extrasystole. The intervals between the normal complexes are the same (x). The extrasystole in this situation is said to be *interpolated.*

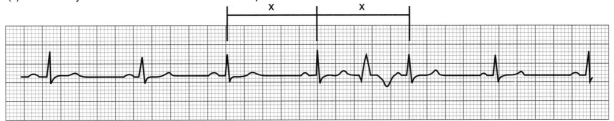

Lead II—normal sinus rhythm with ventricular bigeminy. There is a fixed coupling interval (x) between the normal complexes and the extrasystoles. This strongly supports reentry as the mechanism of the arrhythmia.

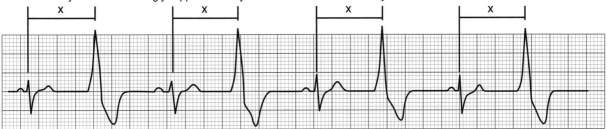

Lead II—normal sinus rhythm with ventricular bigeminy. There are two extrasystoles following the first normal complex.

Lead II—normal sinus rhythm with two multiform ventricular extrasystoles. The mechanism of these complexes is unclear from this strip.

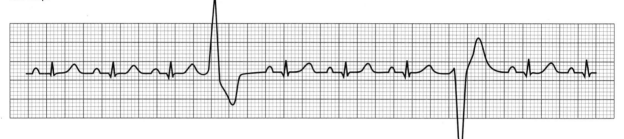

Lead II—normal sinus rhythm with a single ventricular extrasystole. The extrasystole does not reset the atrial rate (the P waves are indicated by vertical lines), but the next two PR intervals (arrows) are prolonged. This is an example of *concealed retrograde conduction*. The extrasystole has depolarized the AV node in a retrograde manner. The next atrial impulse thus finds the AV node partly refractory and the PR interval is prolonged.

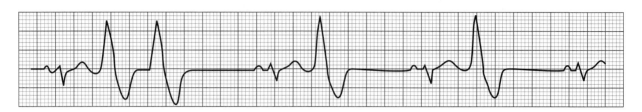

Lead II—the underlying rhythm is atrial fibrillation. There are ventricular extrasystoles which do not have a fixed coupling interval with the normal complexes, but have a constant interval between them. This is an example of *ventricular parasystole*, and usually represents an ectopic mechanism.

X   X   X

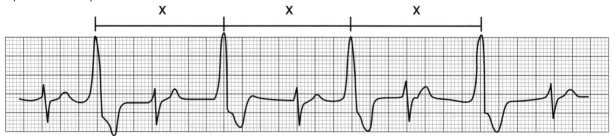

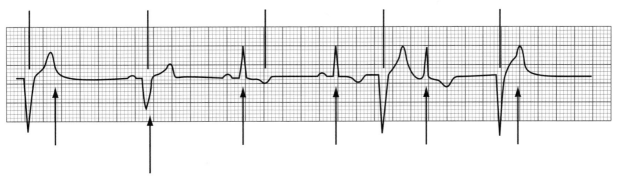

Lead II—sinus rhythm with ventricular parasystole. The lack of a fixed coupling interval suggests an ectopic mechanism. There are independent rates for the sinus complexes (arrows) and the ventricular complexes (vertical lines). The source that depolarizes the ventricle depends on the timing of the two mechanisms. The second complex in the strip is a fusion beat.

II. Preexcitation

   A. The origin of accessory pathways
       1. *In utero*, the atria and ventricles are eventually separated by a fibrous plate called the AV ring.
       2. The function of the AV ring is to provide support for the mitral and tricuspid valves and to electrically insulate the atria and ventricles.
       3. The AV node is the only structure which should allow conduction through the AV ring.
       4. Excessive separation of the atria and ventricles produces congenital third degree AV block (see Day 4).
       5. If there is incomplete separation, residual muscle fibers may bridge the AV ring and form accessory electrical pathways.

   B. Characteristics of accessory pathways
       1. Accessory pathways usually do not have the conduction delay properties of the AV node.
       2. Another way of saying this is that the refractory period of the accessory pathway is typically shorter than the AV node.
       3. Accessory pathways can be located anywhere around the AV ring, and may be multiple.

   C. ECG manifestations of accessory pathways
       1. The delta wave
           a. After atrial systole, the shorter refractory period of the accessory pathway may produce an early depolarization of part of the right or left ventricle.
           b. The early depolarization of part of the ventricle causes the QRS complex to intrude into the PR interval producing the characteristic delta wave.
           c. The location of the delta wave helps localize the site of the accessory pathway.
           d. The presence of the delta wave and its attendant arrhythmias is known as the Wolff-Parkinson-White (WPW) syndrome.

2. Limitations to ECG interpretation
    a. The delta wave may be inverted in various leads and may appear as a Q wave, producing a pseudoinfarct pattern.
    b. QRS voltage is an unreliable indicator of LVH.
    c. ST and T wave changes are unreliable indicators of ischemia unless serial ECGs are available.

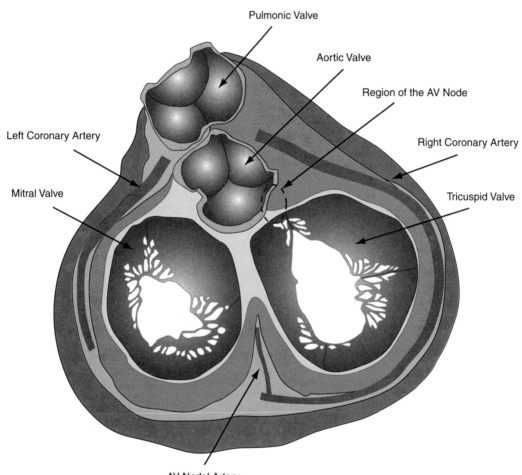

The heart in diastole as viewed from above with the atria removed. The AV ring is a fibrous structure which supports the mitral and tricuspid valves. It also serves as an insulating plate between the atria and ventricles. The AV node is normally the only electrical connection between the atria and ventricles. Accessory pathways are residual muscle fibers which may occur anywhere around the periphery of the AV ring. These pathways may result in the Wolff-Parkinson-White syndrome.

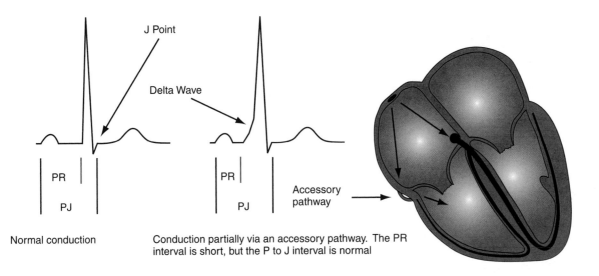

J Point

Delta Wave

PR

PJ

PR

PJ

Accessory
pathway

Normal conduction

Conduction partially via an accessory pathway. The PR
interval is short, but the P to J interval is normal

The ECG complex in WPW with partial conduction down an accessory pathway. The portion of the ventricle which is depolarized early produces the characteristic delta wave and shortens the PR interval.

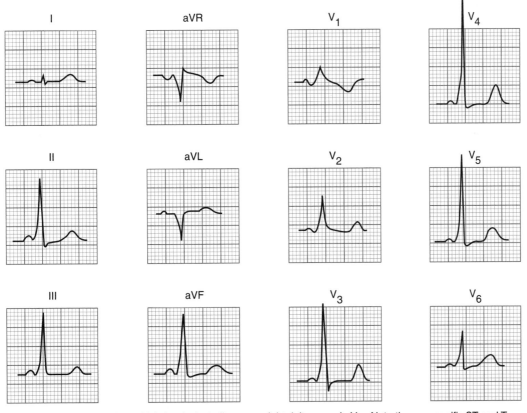

WPW with a delta wave in multiple leads, including an upright delta wave in V_1. Note the nonspecific ST and T wave changes.

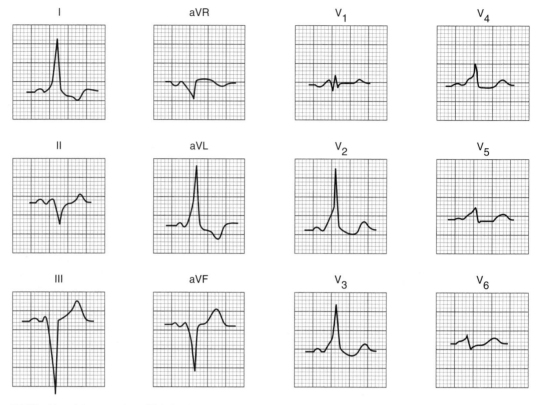

WPW with a delta wave in multiple leads, including a pseudoinfarction pattern in II, III, and aVF.

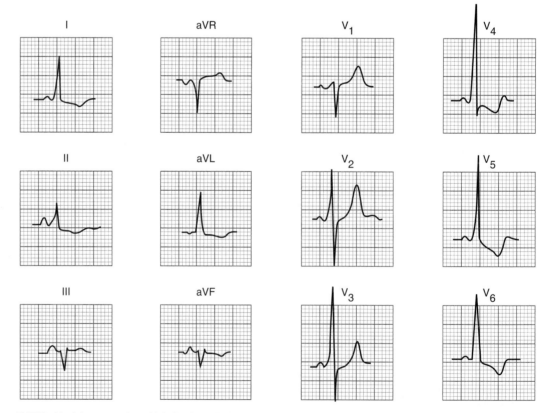

WPW with delta waves in multiple leads, including tall R waves in V_2. Although there are prominent voltages in the chest leads, LVH should not be diagnosed.

D. Accessory pathways and arrhythmias
   1. Reentrant arrhythmias involving an accessory pathway
      a. The accessory pathway may form one limb of a reentrant loop, with the AV node as the other limb.
      b. A reentrant arrhythmia can occur with the wave of depolarization going down the AV node and retrograde up the accessory pathway (antegrade conduction).
      c. As long as there is no concomitant IVCD, the QRS complex with antegrade conduction down the AV node will be narrow (no delta wave).
      d. If the depolarization proceeds down the accessory pathway and back up through the AV node (retrograde conduction), the QRS complex will be wide (and resemble VT).
      e. Maneuvers or medications which block the AV node may terminate these arrhythmias (but see below).
      f. These arrhythmias are known as reciprocating tachycardias.
   2. Atrial fibrillation and atrial flutter with an accessory pathway
      a. If atrial fibrillation or flutter occurs in the presence of an accessory pathway, many impulses may be conducted through the pathway so that the ventricular response is very rapid.
      b. The QRS complex is usually wide and bizarre, and may be irregular if atrial fibrillation is present.
      c. Interventions which increase AV nodal block may speed conduction through the accessory pathway and are contraindicated.
      d. These arrhythmias should be treated with urgent electrical cardioversion and subsequent ablation of the accessory pathway.

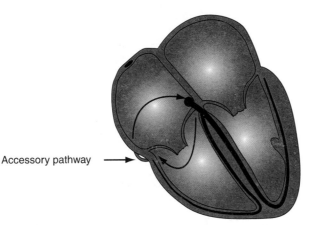

Accessory pathway ⟶

Lead II—a reentrant arrhythmia resulting from antegrade conduction down the AV node and retrograde up the accessory pathway. Note the narrow QRS complexes.

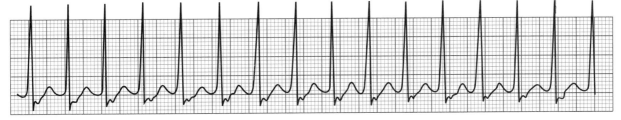

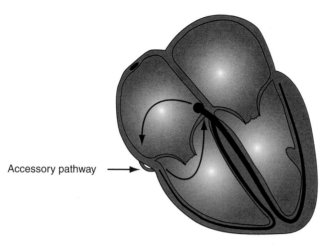

Accessory pathway

Lead II—wide QRS tachycardia resulting from antegrade conduction down an accessory pathway and retrograde return through the AV node.

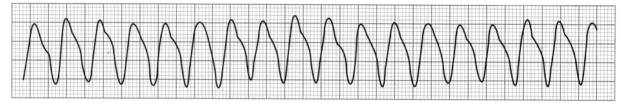

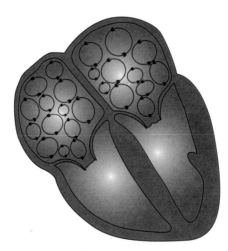

Lead II—atrial fibrillation with rapid conduction down an accessory pathway. Note the wide, rapid, irregular QRS complexes. An occasional normal complex represents competitive conduction through the AV node. This arrhythmia is a medical emergency requiring defibrillation.

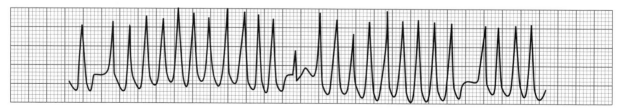

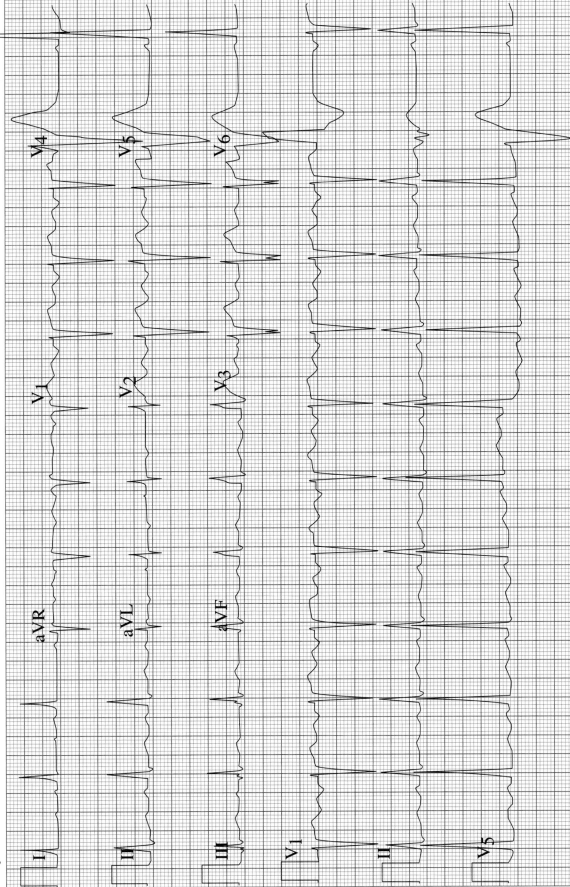

Day 7 ECG 1

Day 7 ECG 2

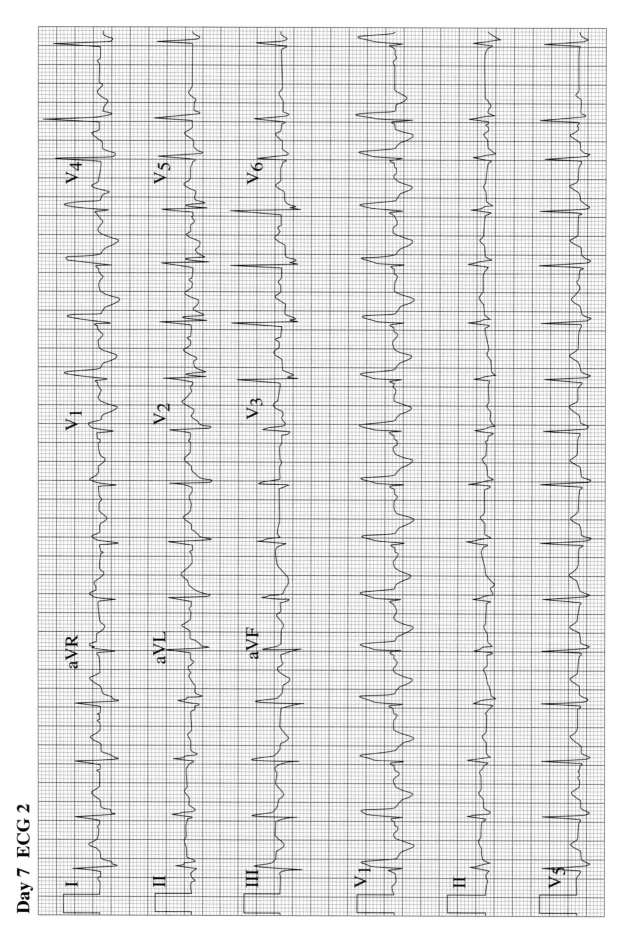

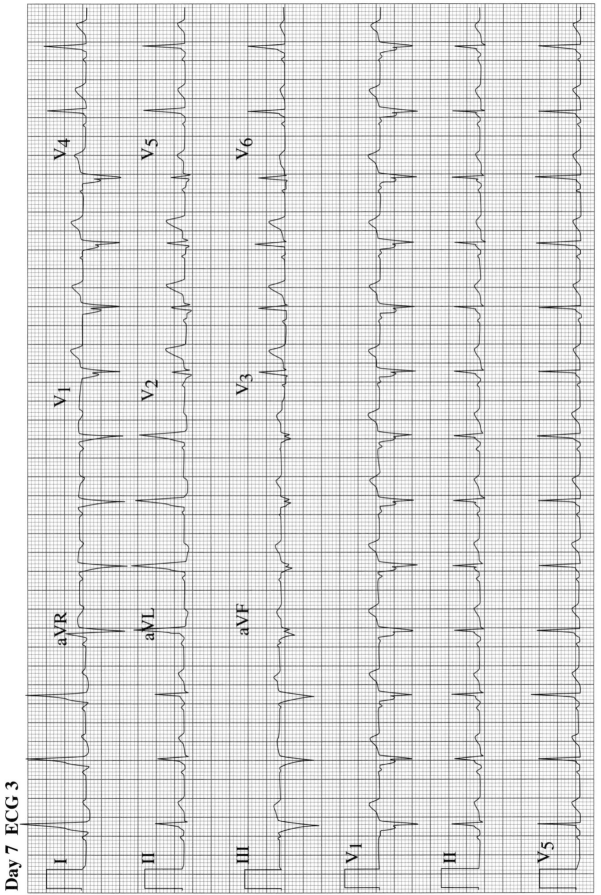

Day 7 ECG 4

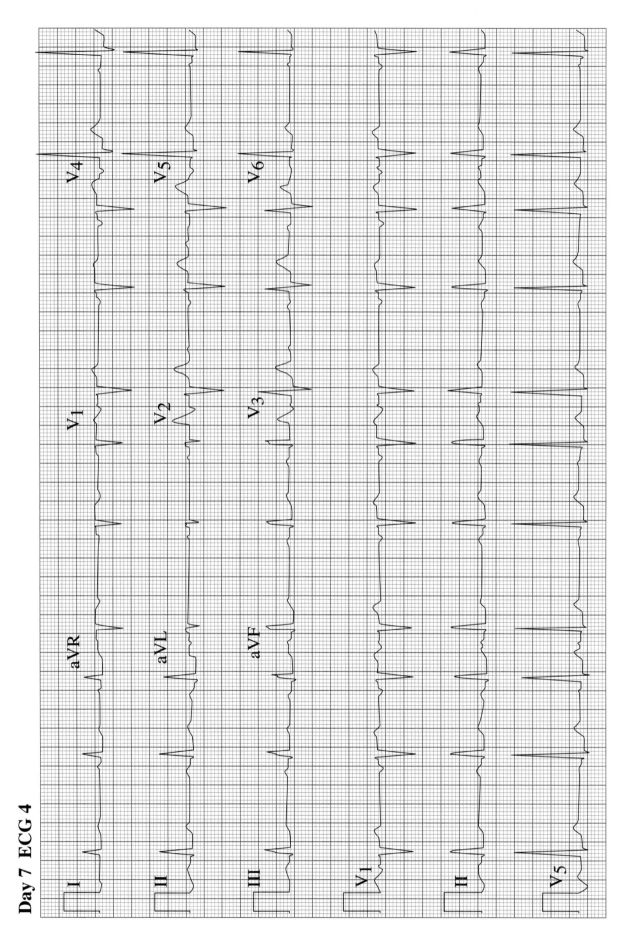

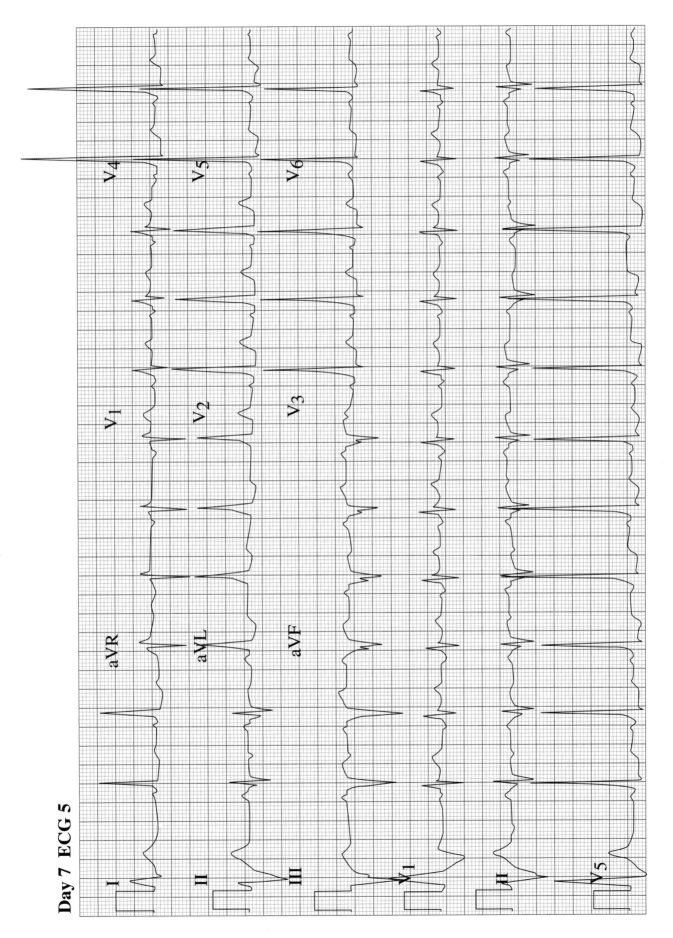

Day 7 ECG 5

179

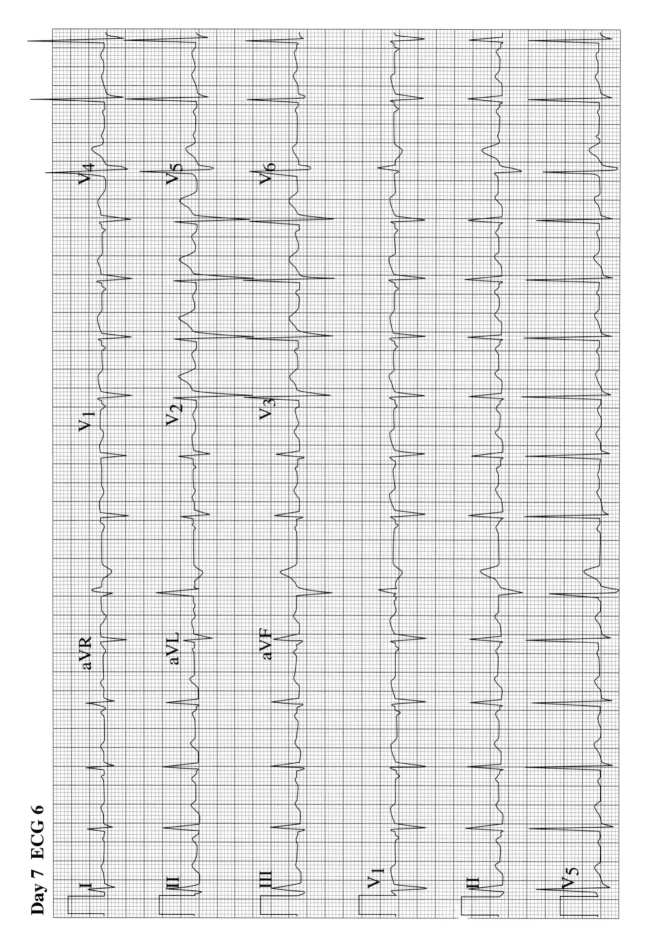

Day 7 ECG 6

180

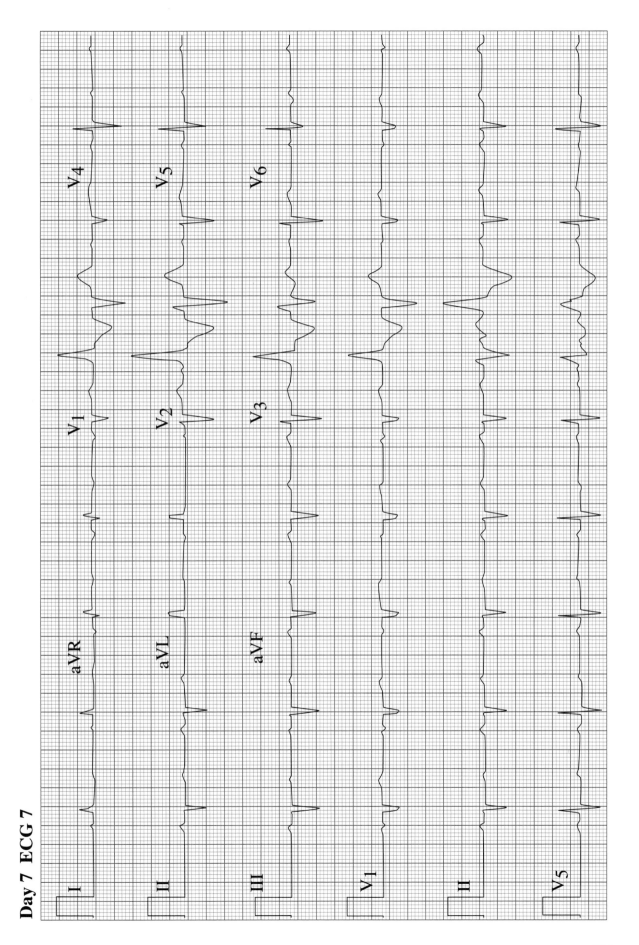

Day 7 ECG 7

I

II

III

V1

II

V5

aVR

aVL

aVF

V1

V2

V3

V4

V5

V6

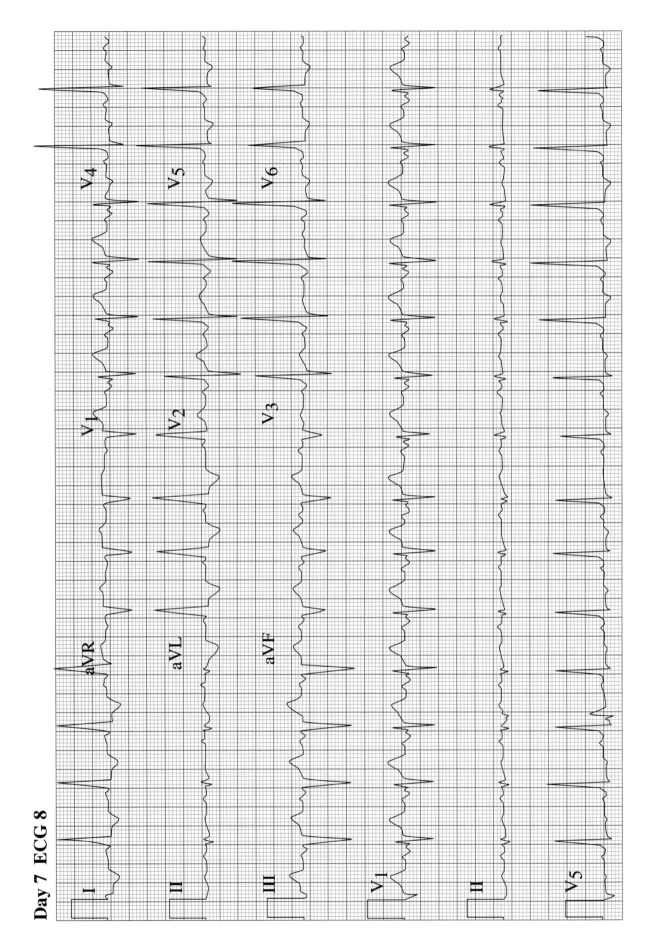

I

II

III

aVR

aVL

aVF

V1

V2

V3

V4

V5

V6

V1

II

V5

Day 7 ECG 9

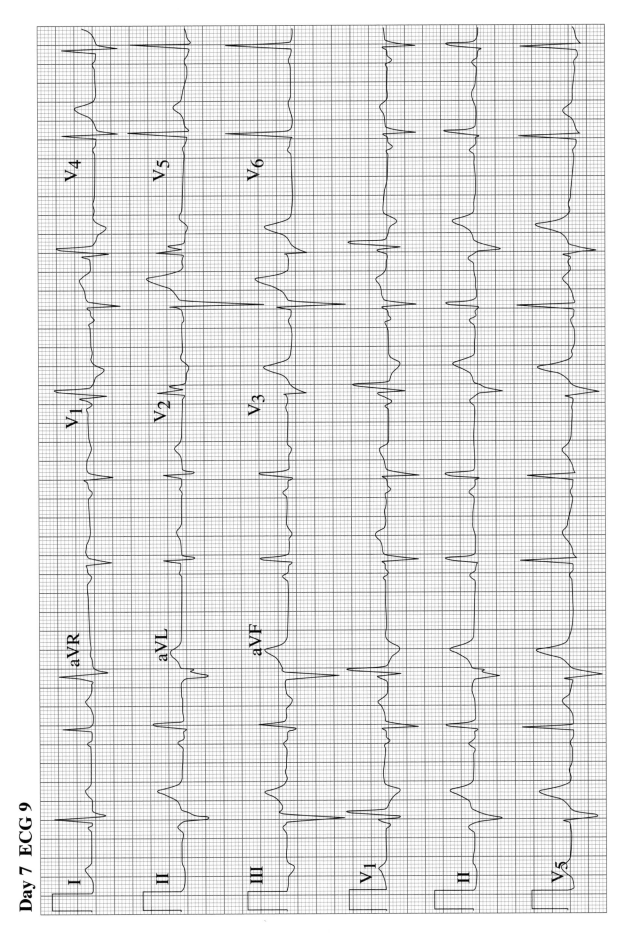

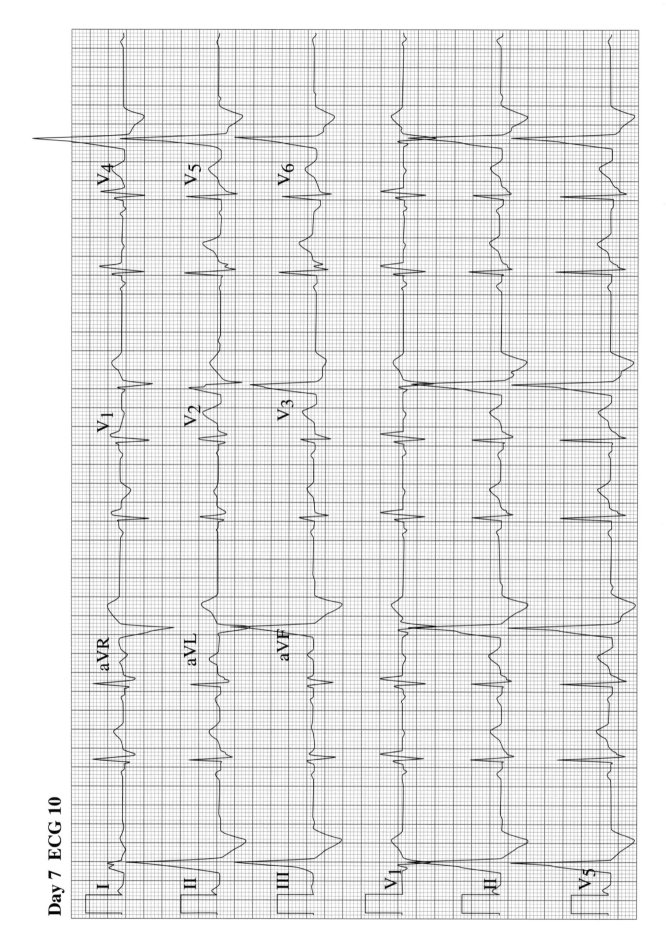

Day 7 ECG 10

184

Day 7
ECG Interpretations and Discussion

Day 7 ECG 1
    Normal sinus rhythm
    Ventricular extrasystoles
    Left atrial abnormality

There is a wide QRS complex which is early and is followed by a compensatory pause, indicating a ventricular extrasystole.

Day 7 ECG 2
    Sinus tachycardia with atrial extrasystoles
    Right bundle branch block
    Inferior MI, age undetermined

There is a QRS complex in the latter part of the ECG which is early. It has the same morphology as the other complexes. There is a deformation of the preceding T wave which probably represents a superimposed P wave. These findings indicate an atrial extrasystole. There is also right bundle branch block and Q waves in the inferior leads consistent with a previous infarct.

Day 7 ECG 3
    Normal sinus rhythm
    Wolff-Parkinson-White syndrome

The PR interval is short and there are obvious delta waves in several leads. There are Q waves in III and aVF which should not be interpreted as an inferior infarct. There are also voltage criteria for left ventricular hypertrophy in I, but, again, this diagnosis cannot be made in the presence of the Wolff-Parkinson-White syndrome.

Day 7 ECG 4
    Normal sinus rhythm with frequent atrial extrasystoles
    Nonspecific ST abnormality

There are frequent early narrow complexes which are preceded by P waves with different morphologies. These represent atrial extrasystoles.

Day 7 ECG 5
    Normal sinus rhythm with occasional ventricular extrasystoles
    Wolff-Parkinson-White syndrome

The PR interval is short and there are obvious delta waves in several leads. There are Q waves in III and aVF which should not be interpreted as an inferior infarct. There is a tall R wave in V_1 which represents an upright delta wave. There are also voltage criteria for left ventricular hypertrophy in I, but, again, this diagnosis cannot be made in the presence of the Wolff-Parkinson-White syndrome.

Day 7 ECG 6
  Normal sinus rhythm with frequent atrial extrasystoles with aberrant conduction

There are early wide complex beats which are preceded by P waves, indicating that these are atrial extrasystoles with aberrant conduction.

Day 7 ECG 7
  Sinus bradycardia with frequent ventricular extrasystoles
  First degree AV block
  Left axis deviation
  Possible inferior MI, age undetermined
  Nonspecific ST and T wave changes

There are frequent wide complexes with different morphologies, consistent with ventricular extrasystoles. The PR interval is greater than 200 msec. There are tiny R waves in the inferior leads, but there still may have been a previous infarct.

Day 7 ECG 8
  Normal sinus rhythm
  Left atrial abnormality
  Wolff-Parkinson-White syndrome

The PR interval is short and there are obvious delta waves in several leads.

Day 7 ECG 9
  Normal sinus rhythm with ventricular parasystole
  Left atrial abnormality
  Nonspecific ST abnormalities

There is sinus rhythm with a competing ventricular ectopic focus, a situation called *ventricular parasystole*. The wide complexes only appear when the ventricle is not already affected by normal activity. The key to recognizing this very uncommon arrhythmia is that the ventricular extrasystoles do not have a fixed coupling interval to the previous normal beats. Almost all ventricular extrasystoles of similar morphology do have a fixed coupling interval, demonstrating their reentrant etiology. The next step is to identify a constant interval between the extrasystoles. Since this is a ventricular arrhythmia, the rate is typically 20–40. There may be long gaps between the extrasystoles since they have to compete with the regular rhythm.

Day 7 ECG 10
  Normal sinus rhythm with frequent ventricular extrasystoles
  Right bundle branch block

There are frequent wide complexes with a similar morphology and a fixed coupling interval to the preceding normal beats. This is the typical presentation of reentrant ventricular extrasystoles. This situation is many times more common than the preceding example.

Day 8

The Differential Diagnosis of Wide QRS Tachycardias

I. Basic considerations

 A. Wide QRS tachycardias represent either VT or SVT with aberrant conduction.

 B. VT and SVT represent vastly different clinical situations as far as etiology, extent of underlying cardiac disease, treatment, and prognosis.

 C. The following discussion applies to hemodynamically stable patients; unstable patients should have emergent electrocardioversion.

II. Brugada's criteria

 A. In 1991, Brugada published a landmark paper on this problem, and his algorithm will be followed here [Brugada P, et al, A new approach to the differential diagnosis of a regular tachycardia with a wide QRS complex. *Circulation*, 1991;83(5):1649–1659].

 B. Brugada's criteria are based on the standard 12-lead ECG, but additional leads and techniques may aid in diagnosis.

III. Application of Brugada's criteria (see tree diagram)

 A. The presence and duration of an RS complex in the precordial leads
  1. Any initial R wave followed by an S wave in the precordial leads qualifies for analysis.
  2. Lack of an RS in any precordial lead is highly specific for VT.
  3. An RS interval (defined as the interval between the onset of the R wave and the nadir of the S wave in any precordial lead) greater than 100 msec is highly specific for VT.

 B. AV dissociation
  1. The presence of AV dissociation is highly specific for VT.
  2. AV dissociation can be detected on the standard ECG in about 20% of VT.

3. Methods for detection of AV dissociation
    a. Examination of the patient may reveal irregular cannon A waves in the neck veins caused by coincidental simultaneous atrial and ventricular systole.
    b. Standard ECG leads II, III, aVF, and V_2 are best for detecting P waves.
    c. Moving one of the chest leads to the V_3R position may reveal P waves.
    d. An S_5 or "Lewis' leads" is obtained by placing the right arm lead in the second right interspace and the left arm lead in the suprasternal notch with the ECG machine set to Lead I.
    e. A transesophageal or intraatrial lead may be necessary to make a definitive diagnosis.

C. The morphology of the QRS complexes in V_{1-2} and V_6 (see morphology criteria table below)
    1. The first determination is whether the QRS morphology in the precordial leads is a RBBB or a LBBB.
    2. If the QRS complexes in V_{1-2} and V_6 both meet criteria for VT (see diagram following table), VT is confirmed.
    3. If there is discordance between the criteria for VT in V_{1-2} and V_6, SVT is strongly implicated.

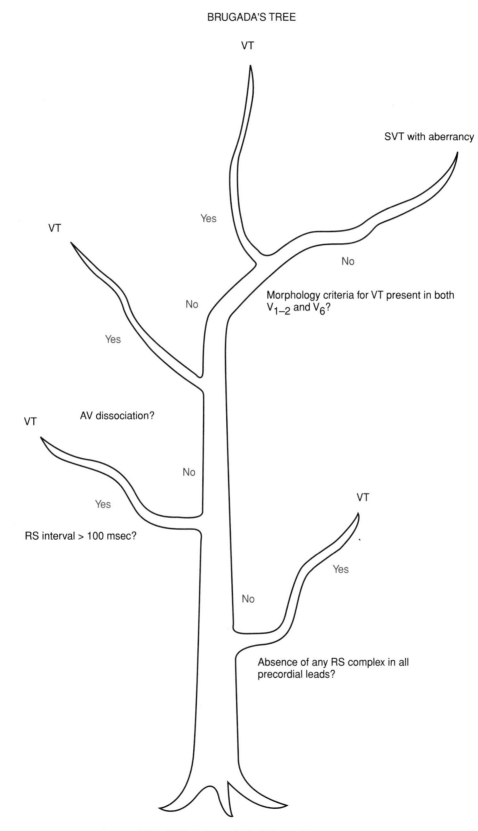

BRUGADA'S TREE

Wide QRS tachycardia (> 120 msec)

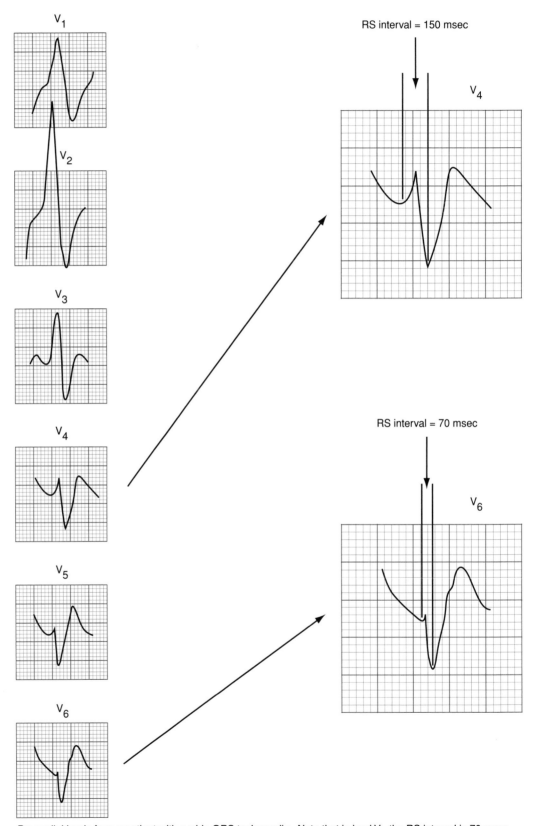

Precordial leads from a patient with a wide QRS tachycardia. Note that in lead V_6 the RS interval is 70 msec, but in V_4 the interval is 160 msec, confirming that this arrhythmia is VT.

Morphology Criteria for VT versus SVT

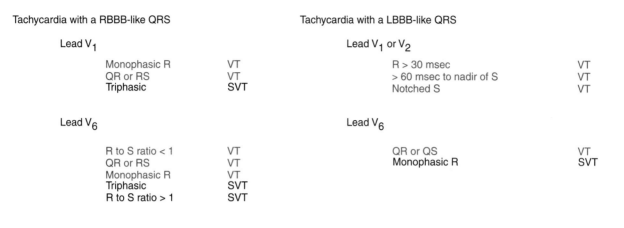

Tachycardia with a RBBB-like QRS			Tachycardia with a LBBB-like QRS		
Lead V₁			**Lead V₁ or V₂**		
Monophasic R	VT		R > 30 msec	VT	
QR or RS	VT		> 60 msec to nadir of S	VT	
Triphasic	SVT		Notched S	VT	
Lead V₆			**Lead V₆**		
R to S ratio < 1	VT		QR or QS	VT	
QR or RS	VT		Monophasic R	SVT	
Monophasic R	VT				
Triphasic	SVT				
R to S ratio > 1	SVT				

Examples of Morphology Criteria with RBBB-like QRS complexes

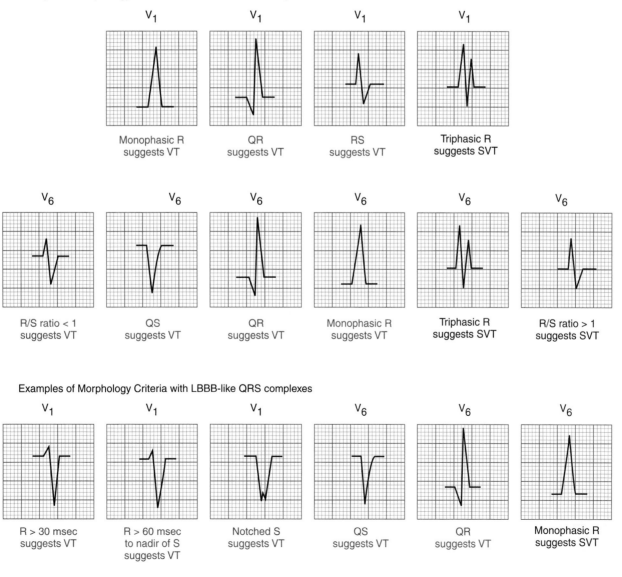

Examples of Morphology Criteria with LBBB-like QRS complexes

Lead V$_1$

Lead V$_4$

Lead V$_2$

Lead V$_5$

Lead V$_3$

Lead V$_6$

Lead V$_1$

Lead II

Lead V$_5$

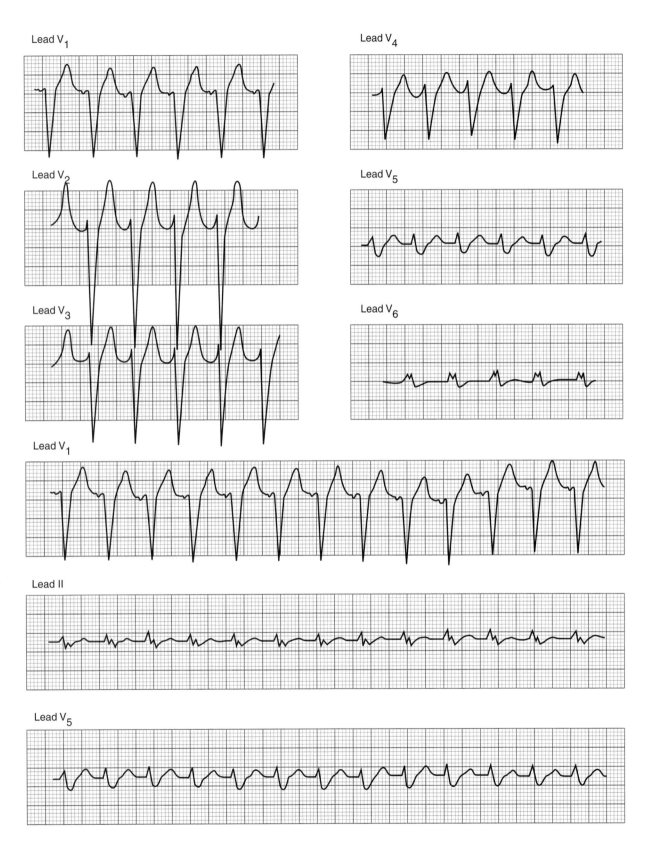

Example 1—a wide QRS tachycardia of the LBBB type which has RS complexes in the precordial leads. The RS interval is less than 100 msec and tiny P waves can be detected in V$_1$. This is sinus tachycardia with nonspecific IVCD (not quite a LBBB).

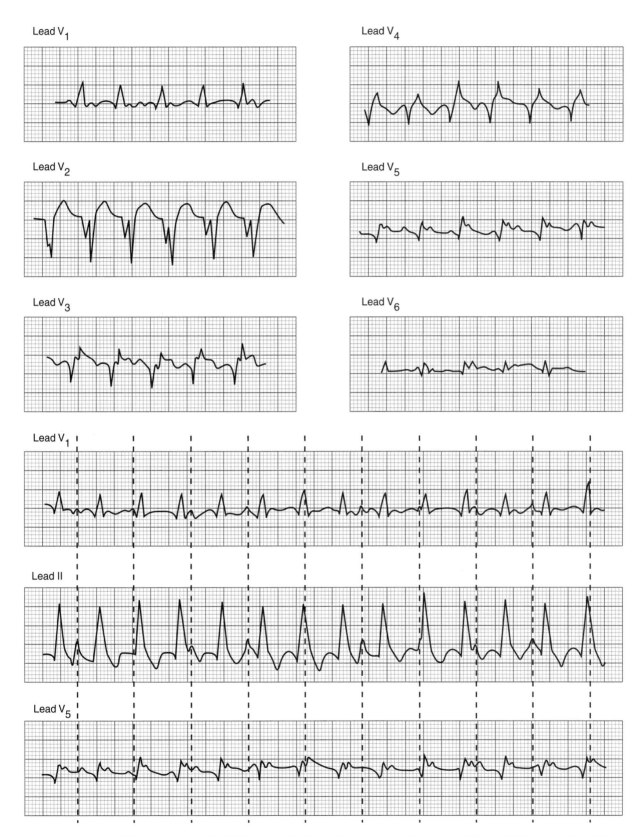

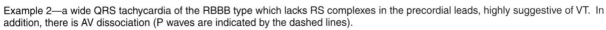

Example 2—a wide QRS tachycardia of the RBBB type which lacks RS complexes in the precordial leads, highly suggestive of VT. In addition, there is AV dissociation (P waves are indicated by the dashed lines).

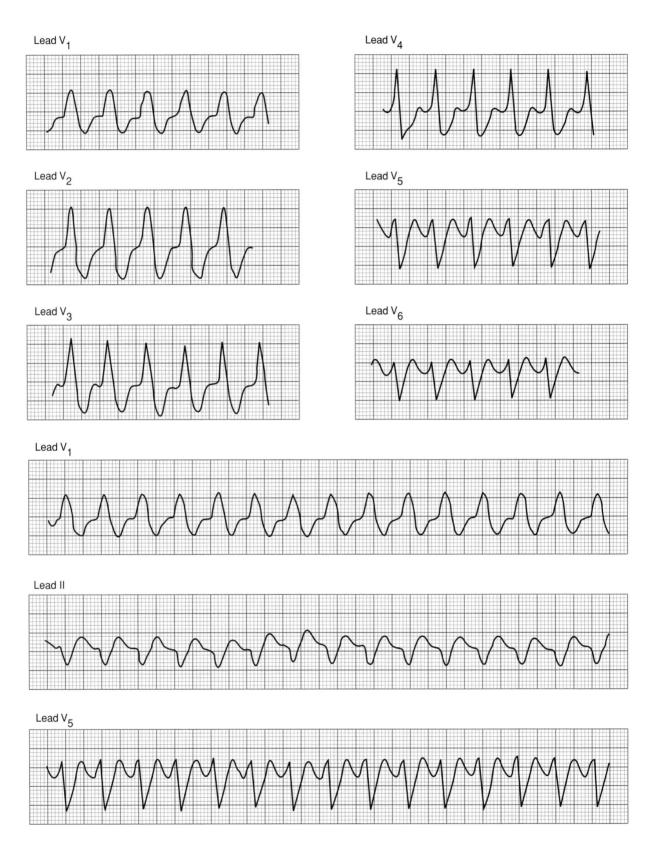

Example 3—a wide QRS tachycardia of the RBBB type which has RS complexes in the precordial leads. The RS interval is greater than 100 msec in several precordial leads, highly suggestive of VT.

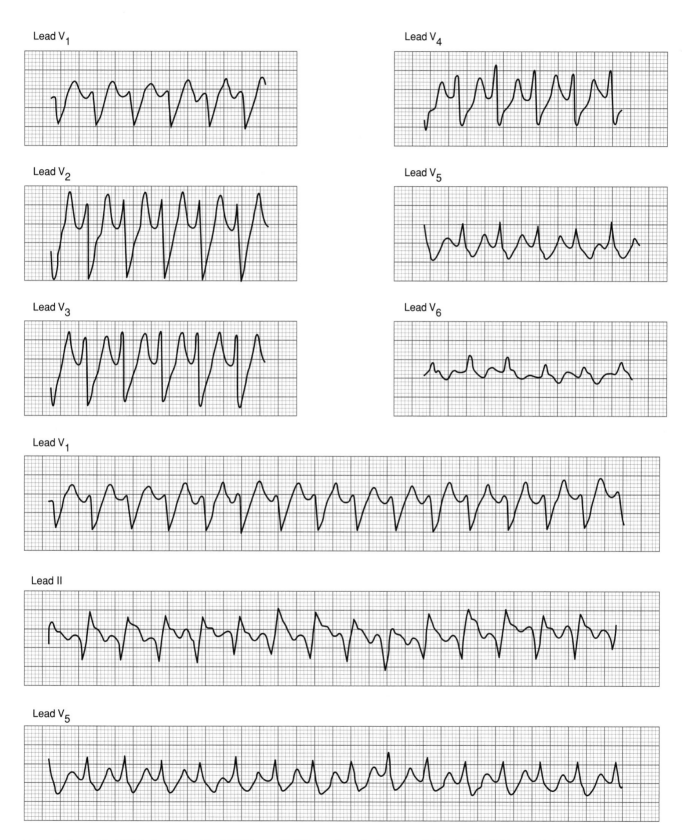

Example 4—a wide QRS tachycardia of the LBBB type with RS complexes in the precordial leads. The RS interval is less than 100 msec. AV dissociation is not apparent. Morphology criteria for VT are present in V_1 but not in V_6, suggesting SVT.

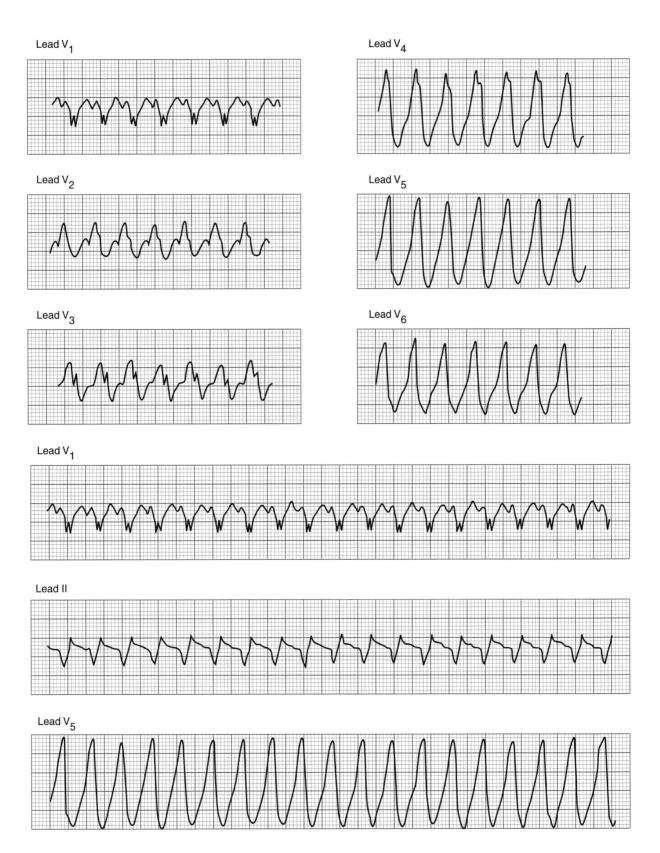

Example 5—a wide QRS tachycardia of the LBBB type with RS complexes in the precordial leads. The RS interval is greater than 100 msec in several leads, consistent with VT.

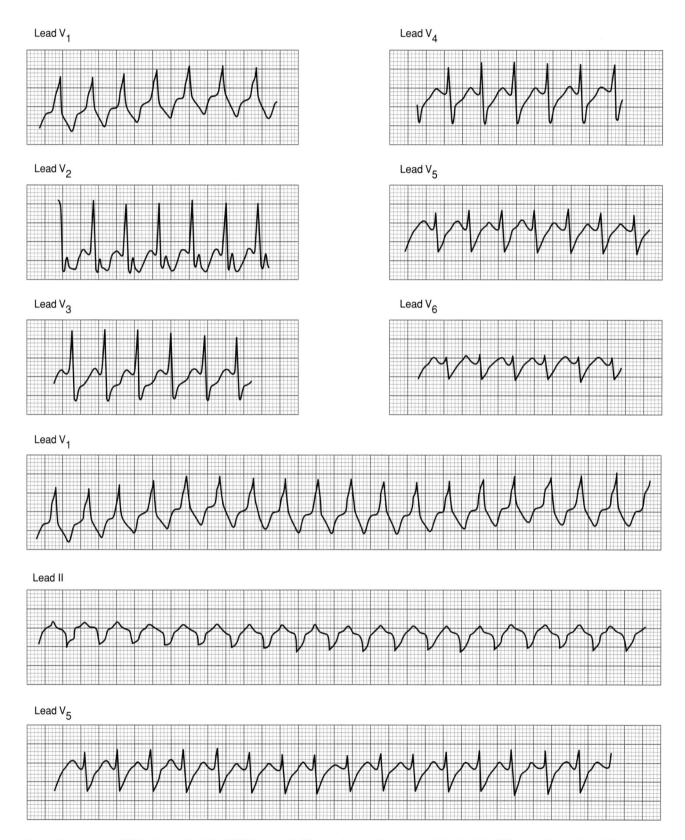

Example 6—a wide QRS tachycardia of the RBBB type with RS complexes in the precordial leads. The RS interval is less than 100 msec. AV dissociation is not apparent. Morphology criteria for VT are present in V_1 and V_6, suggesting VT. However, this arrhythmia was later demonstrated to be PSVT with RBBB, demonstrating that not every arrhythmia can be categorized by 12-lead ECG alone.

Lead V$_4$

Right atrial electrogram

Lead V$_6$

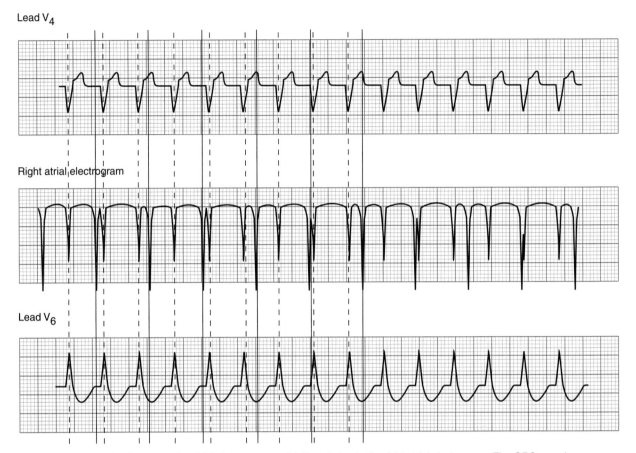

Example 7—a wide QRS tachycardia which demonstrates AV dissociation in the right atrial electrogram. The QRS complexes are indicated by the dashed lines and the P waves by the solid lines. Note that the P waves are larger than the QRS complexes in the atrial electrogram.

Day 8 ECG 1

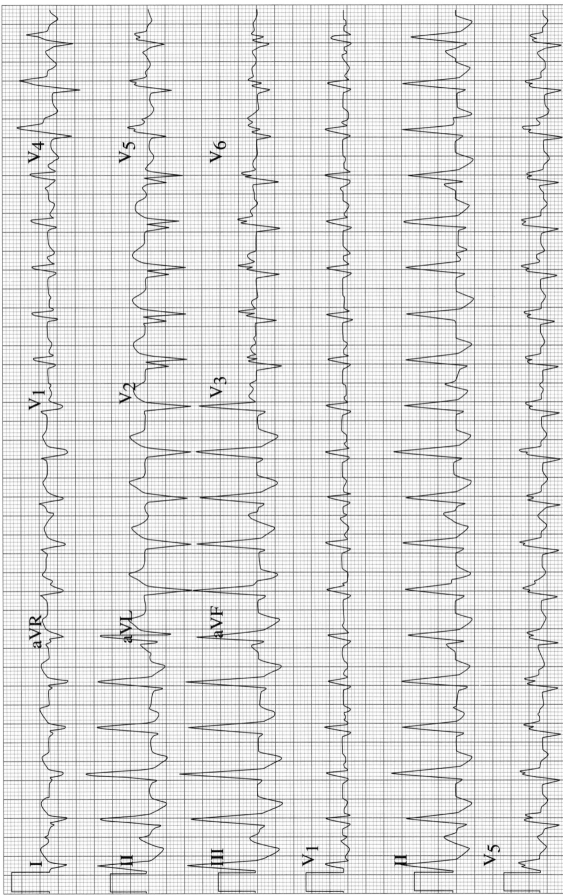

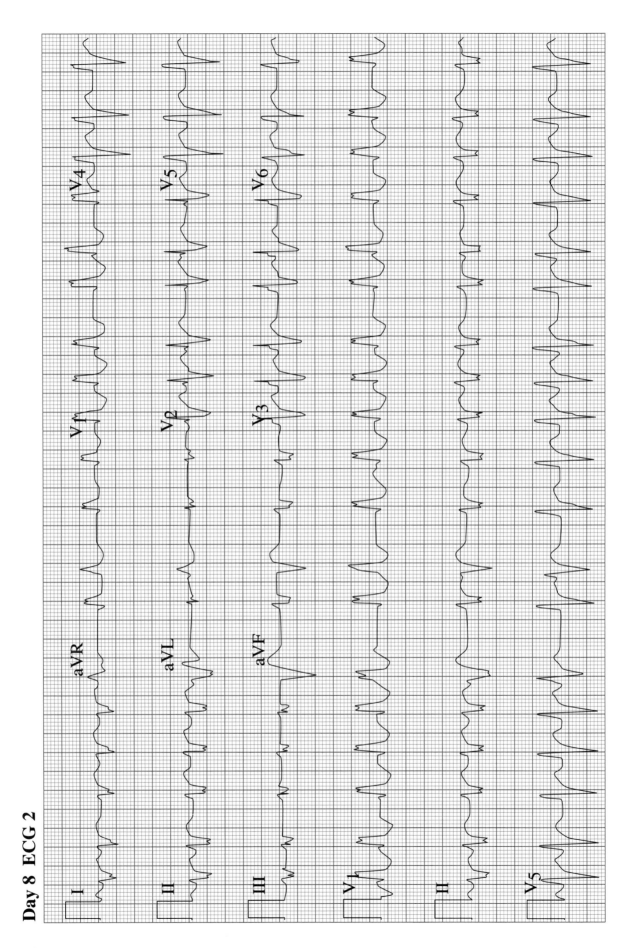

Day 8 ECG 2

200

Day 8 ECG 3

Chest leads are at half standard

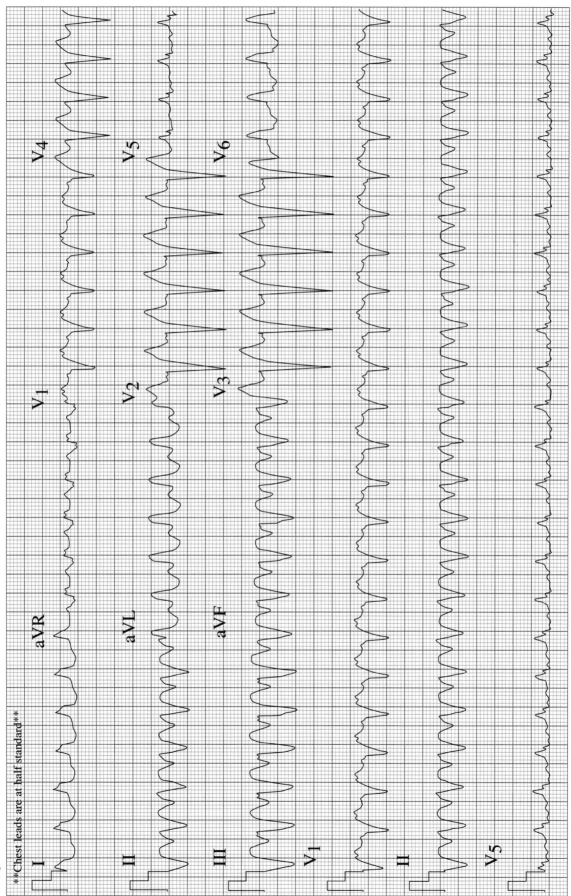

201

Day 8 ECG 4

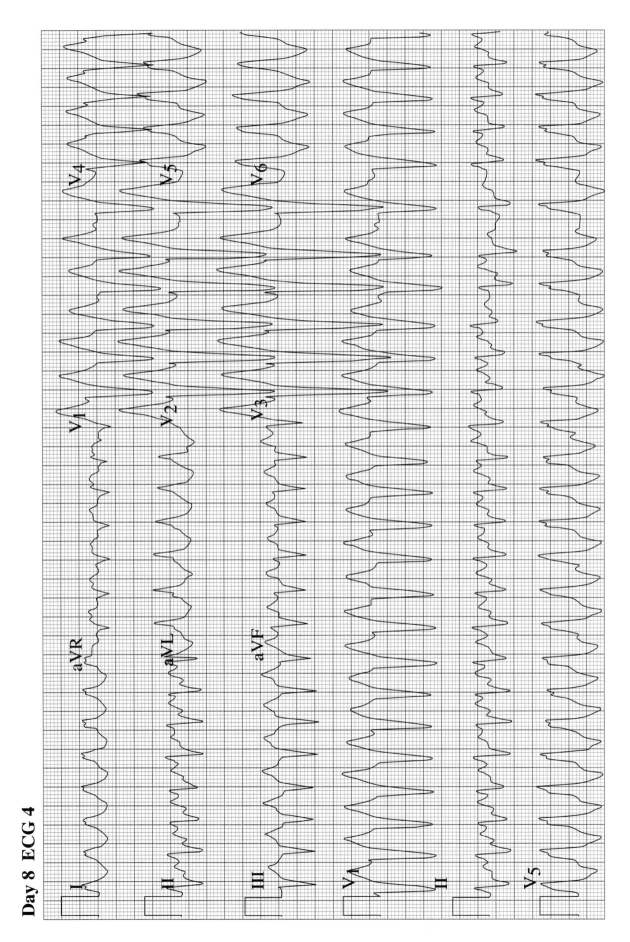

I aVR V1 V4

II aVL V2 V5

III aVF V3 V6

V1

II

V5

Day 8 ECG 5

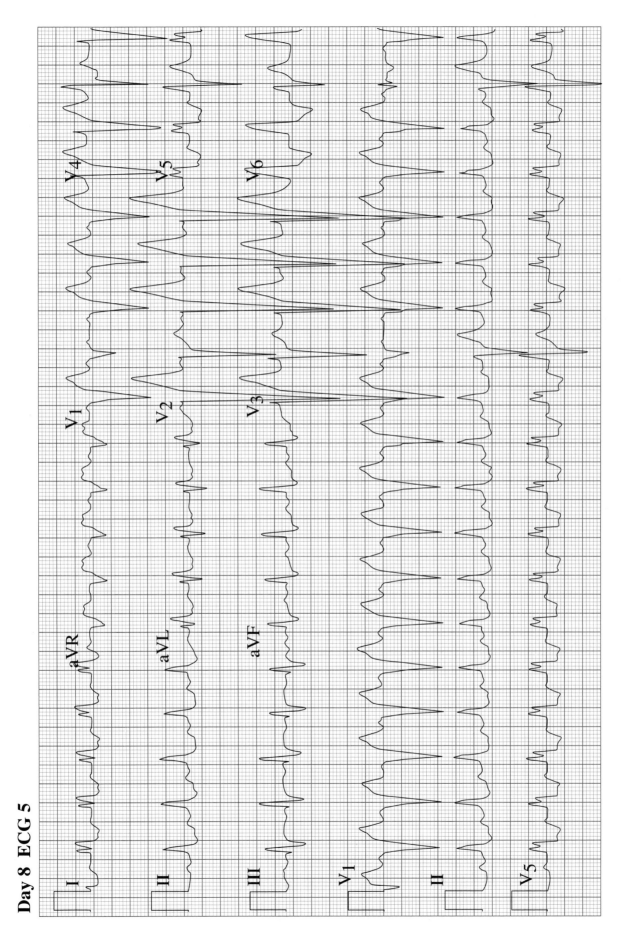

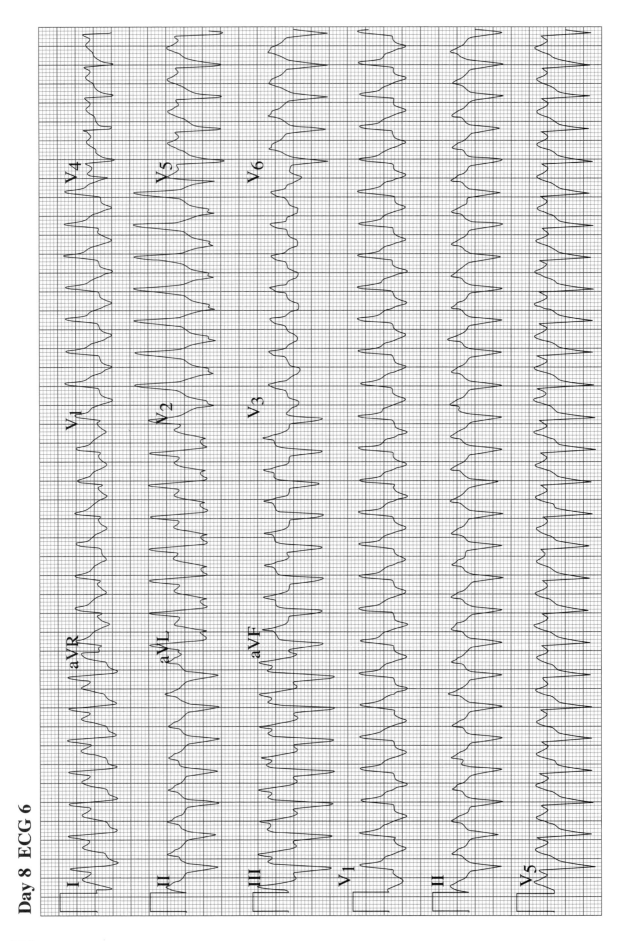

Day 8 ECG 7

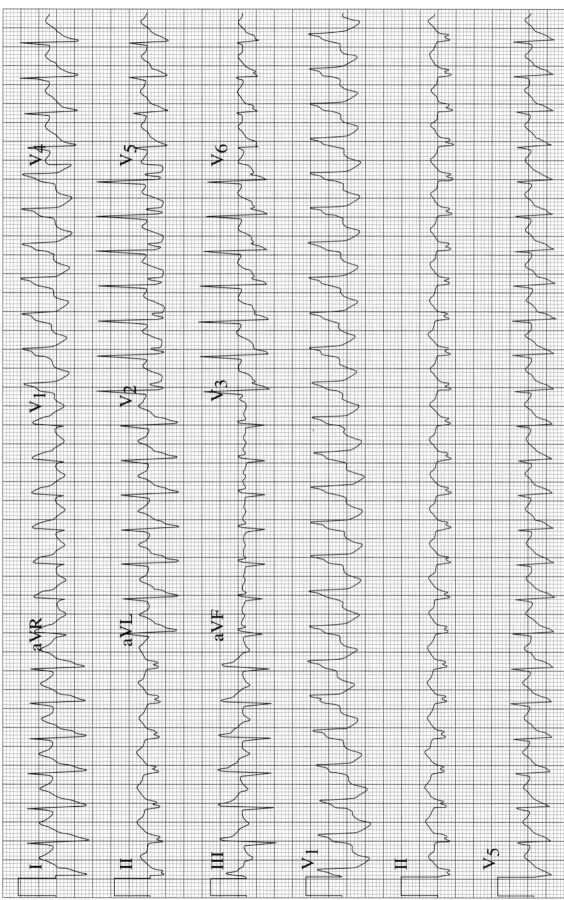

Day 8 ECG 8

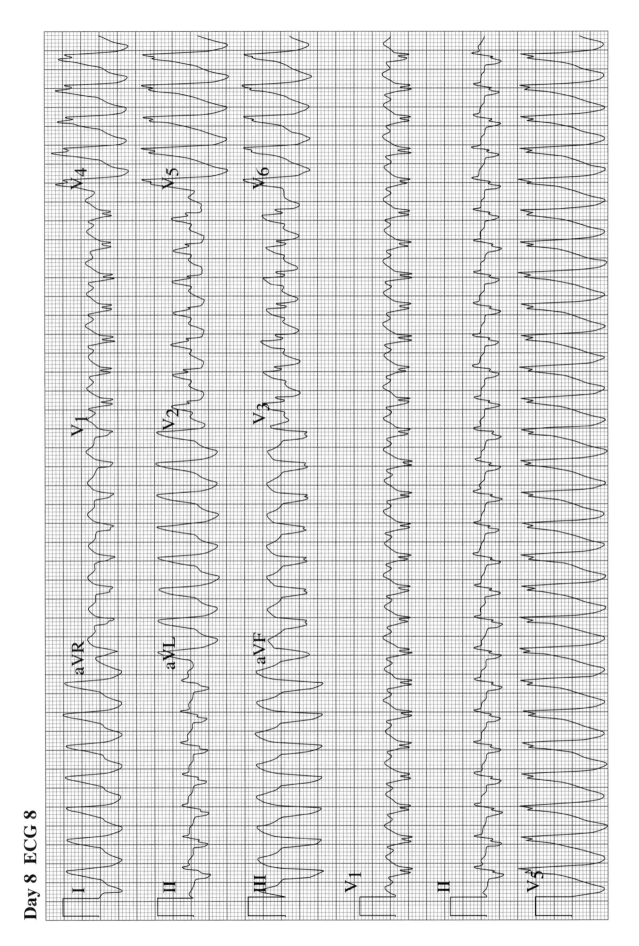

Day 8 ECG 9

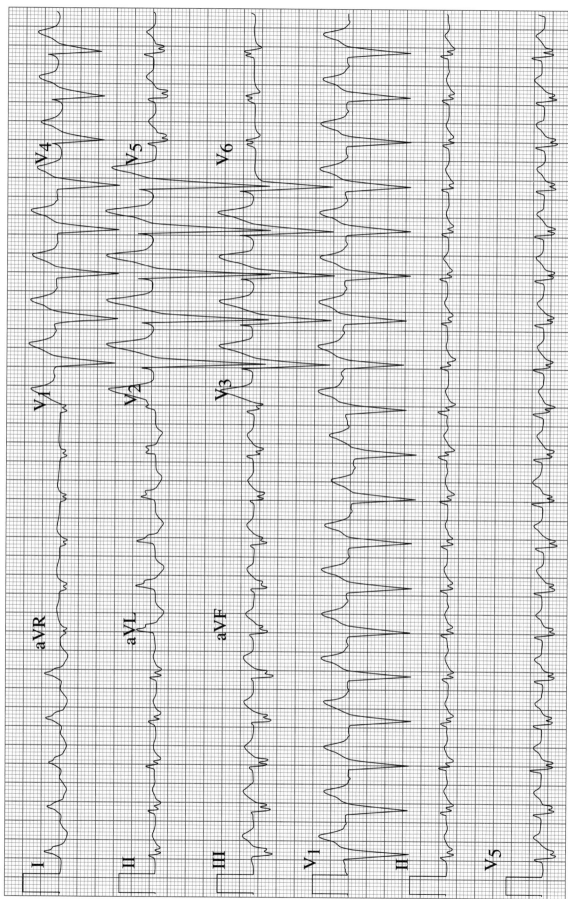

Day 8 ECG 10

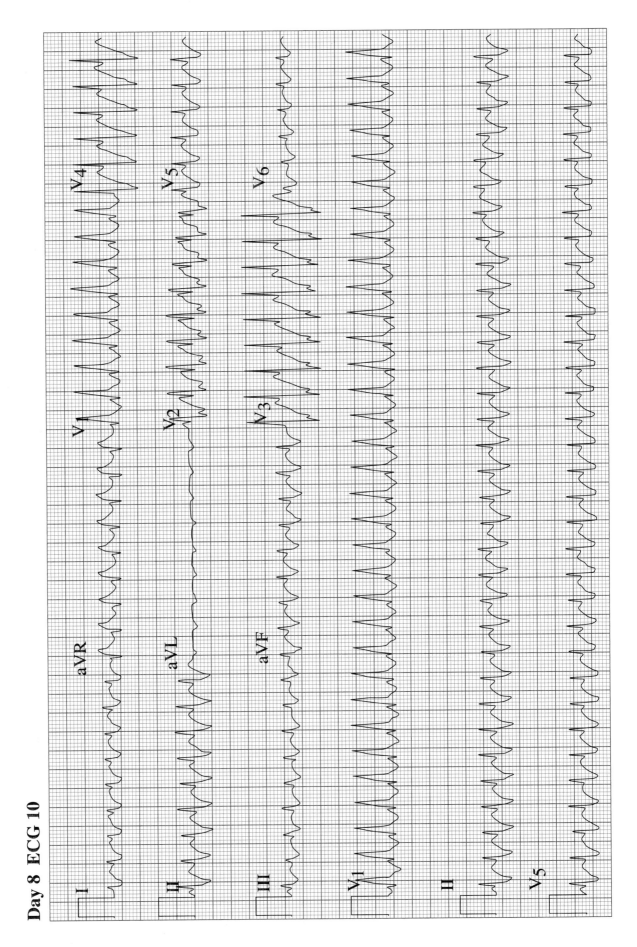

Day 8
ECG Interpretations and Discussion

Day 8 ECG 1

Ventricular tachycardia with underlying sinus rhythm

This is a wide complex tachycardia which has no RS complexes in the precordial leads, consistent with ventricular tachycardia. AV dissociation can also be identified in the V_1 and Lead II rhythm strips.

Day 8 ECG 2

Atrial fibrillation with rapid ventricular response
Right superior axis deviation
Right bundle branch block

This is a wide complex tachycardia which is quite irregular. During longer intervals, an irregular baseline can be detected, indicating atrial fibrillation with right bundle branch block. Using Brugada's criteria, there are RS complexes in the precordial leads, but the RS intervals do not exceed 100 msec, confirming a supraventricular tachycardia.

Day 8 ECG 3

Atrial flutter with 2:1 AV block
Left bundle branch block

This is a wide complex tachycardia which has RS complexes in the precordial leads. The RS intervals do not exceed 100 msec, indicating a supraventricular tachycardia. In addition, regular P waves at a rate of about 280 can be detected in V_1, consistent with atrial flutter with 2:1 AV block and left bundle branch block.

Day 8 ECG 4

Ventricular tachycardia with underlying sinus rhythm

This is a wide complex tachycardia which has RS complexes in the precordial leads. Several of the RS intervals are longer than 100 msec, consistent with ventricular tachycardia. AV dissociation can also be identified in the V_1 and Lead II rhythm strips.

Day 8 ECG 5

Atrial flutter with 2:1 AV block and frequent ventricular extrasystoles
Left bundle branch block

This is a wide complex tachycardia which fortunately has a premature complex about two-thirds across the tracing. This event exposes the baseline (particularly in V_1) long enough to appreciate P waves. The atrial rate is about 260, consistent with atrial flutter with 2:1 AV block, left bundle branch block, and frequent ventricular extrasystoles.

Day 8 ECG 6
   Ventricular tachycardia

This is a wide complex tachycardia which has RS complexes in the precordial leads. Several of the RS intervals are longer than 100 msec, indicating ventricular tachycardia.

Day 8 ECG 7
   PSVT
   Left axis deviation
   Right bundle branch block
   Inferior MI, age undetermined

This is a wide complex tachycardia which has RS complexes in the precordial leads. The RS intervals do not exceed 100 msec, indicating a supraventricular tachycardia. The rate of 150 should raise the possibility of atrial flutter, but this arrhythmia stopped suddenly with vagal maneuvers, indicating PSVT. Once the supraventricular source of this rhythm is established, the additional diagnoses are appropriate.

Day 8 ECG 8
   Ventricular tachycardia

This is a wide complex tachycardia which has RS complexes in the precordial leads. Several of the RS intervals are longer than 100 msec, consistent with ventricular tachycardia.

Day 8 ECG 9
   Sinus tachycardia
   Nonspecific intraventricular conduction defect

This is a wide complex tachycardia, but tiny P waves precede each QRS complex in V_1.

Day 8 ECG 10
   Atrial flutter with 1:1 AV conduction
   Left axis deviation
   Right bundle branch block

This is a very rapid wide complex tachycardia. There are RS complexes in the precordial leads, but none of the RS intervals exceed 100 msec, indicating a supraventricular tachycardia. The rate of 230 is a bit slow for atrial flutter, but this rhythm was confirmed by vagal maneuvers.

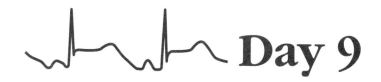 **Day 9**

Medication and Electrolyte Effects; Miscellaneous Conditions

I. Medication effects

A. Digoxin
1. Digoxin has a narrow therapeutic to toxic ratio, and is a potent stimulator of arrhythmias.
2. At therapeutic levels, digoxin frequently causes nonspecific ST changes with "scooping" of the ST segment and shortening of the QT interval.
3. Digoxin causes SA nodal suppression and AV block.
4. Digoxin can cause virtually any arrhythmia, but, because of its ability to enhance automaticity, ectopic arrhythmias are commonly encountered in digoxin toxicity.
5. The commonest arrhythmia manifested by digoxin toxicity is multifocal PVCs.
6. The two most specific arrhythmias are accelerated junctional rhythm and atrial tachycardia with AV block.

Lead II—sinus rhythm with 1st degree AV block, scooping of the ST segments, and a relatively short QT interval consistent with digoxin effect

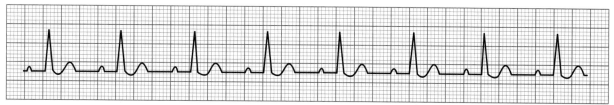

Lead II—sinus rhythm with multiform ventricular extrasystoles

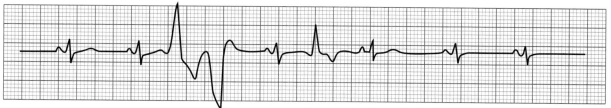

Lead II—accelerated junctional rhythm

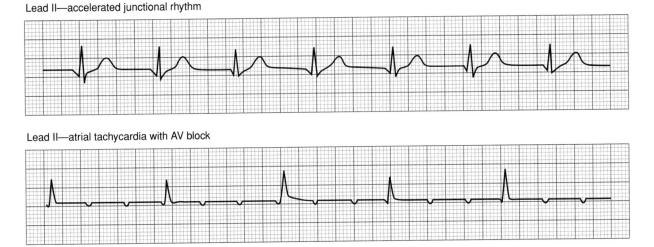

Lead II—atrial tachycardia with AV block

B. Sotalol and amiodarone
  1. These agents slow conduction in general and result in bradycardia and prolongation of the PR, QRS and QT intervals.
  2. Sotalol also has significant beta blocking properties which exacerbate the bradyarrhythmic effects.

Lead II—sinus bradycardia, first degree AV block, a nonspecific IVCD, and QT prolongation in a patient on sotalol

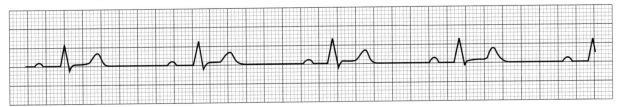

C. Quinidine and other class IA agents (see long QT below)
  1. These agents are less frequently used than previously because of side effects, proarrhythmic potential, and possibly increased mortality.
  2. Quinidine prolongs the QRS duration and QT interval, and may cause torsade de pointes (polymorphic ventricular tachycardia).

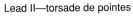

Lead II—torsade de pointes

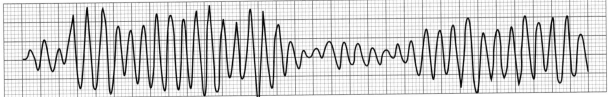

II. Electrolyte abnormalities
  A. Hypokalemia
    1. Hypokalemia potentiates a variety of arrhythmias, including VT and torsade de pointes.
    2. Hypokalemia is associated with ST segment depression and a prominent U wave.

B. Hyperkalemia
1. Hyperkalemia is manifested by peaked T waves and prolongation of the PR segment and QRS duration.
2. When potassium levels reach 8–9 mg/dL, the ECG may resemble a sine wave; further elevation may cause asystole.

Lead V$_5$—ST segment depression and prominent U waves consistent with hypokalemia

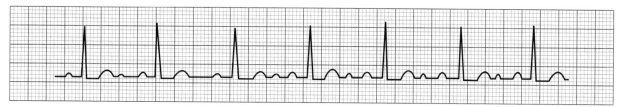

Lead V$_3$—peaked T waves in hyperkalemia (potassium level 7.8 mg/dL)

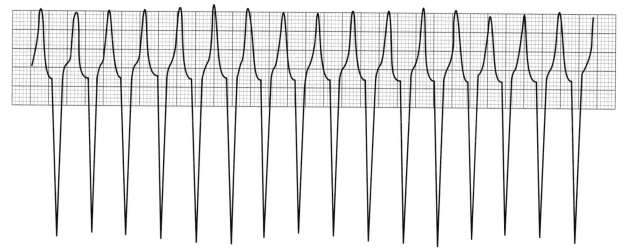

Lead II—PR and QRS prolongation, peaked T waves in hyperkalemia

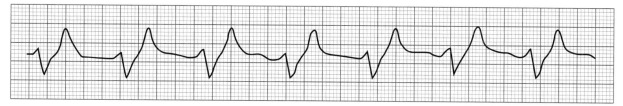

Lead II—deterioration to a sine wave pattern in severe hyperkalemia (9.5 mg/dL)

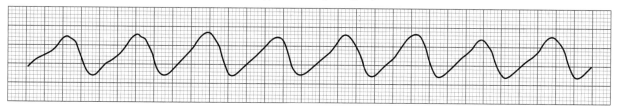

C. Hypocalcemia is manifested by prolongation of the QT interval; the ST segment is usually flat and the T wave is not distorted.

D. Hypercalcemia is associated with a short QT interval.

Lead II—QT prolongation in hypocalcemia

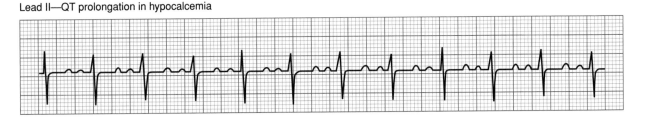

III. QT prolongation and U wave abnormalities

A. A rough indicator of QT prolongation is that the QT interval should not exceed one half of the surrounding R-R interval.

B. Congenital long QT syndromes
    1. There are at least two forms of congenital long QT syndromes:
        a. Jervell and Lange-Nielsen syndrome is an autosomal recessive disorder associated with deafness.
        b. Romano-Ward syndrome is an autosomal dominant disorder.

C. Acquired long QT syndromes
    1. Non-drug causes of long QT interval include ischemia, CNS lesions, and significant bradyarrhythmias.
    2. Drug causes include the Class IA, IC, and III antiarrhythmic agents, erythromycin, and non-sedating antihistamines such as astemizole and terfenedine.

D. U wave abnormalities
    1. Prominent U waves are seen with hypokalemia, digoxin, LVH, and amiodarone.
    2. Negative U waves are encountered in HTN, aortic and mitral disease, and ischemia.

Lead II—long QT interval associated with ischemia

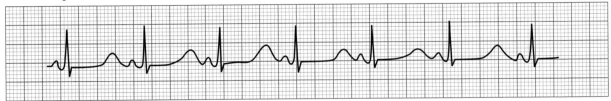

Lead V$_4$—prominent inverted U waves

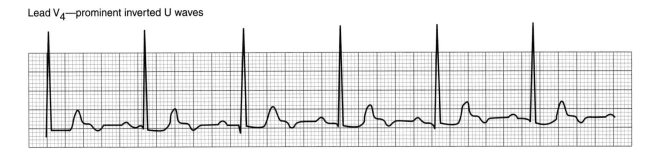

IV. Causes of tall R waves in V$_1$

    A. RVH

    B. Posterior MI

    C. RBBB

    D. WPW

    E. Hypertrophic obstructive cardiomyopathy (HOCM) with asymmetric septal hypertrophy (ASH)

    F. Congenital dextrocardia

    G. Duchenne's muscular dystrophy

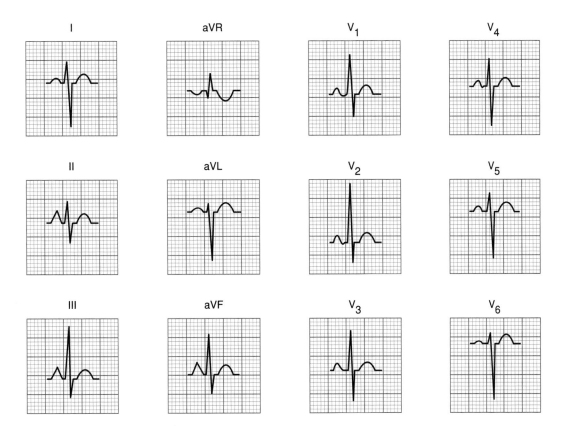

RVH with a tall R wave in V$_1$, right axis deviation, and right atrial abnormality

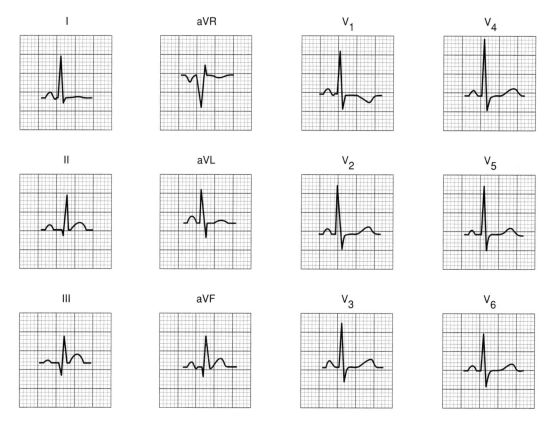

I aVR V₁ V₄

II aVL V₂ V₅

III aVF V₃ V₆

Posterior MI with a tall R wave in V₁ and Q waves in II, III, and aVF

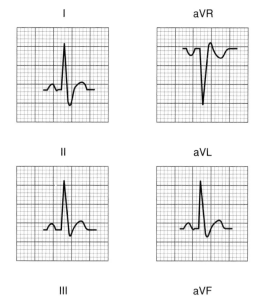
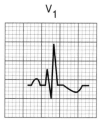
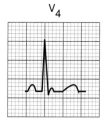
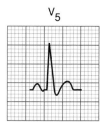
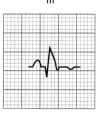
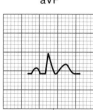
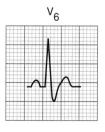

Right bundle branch block

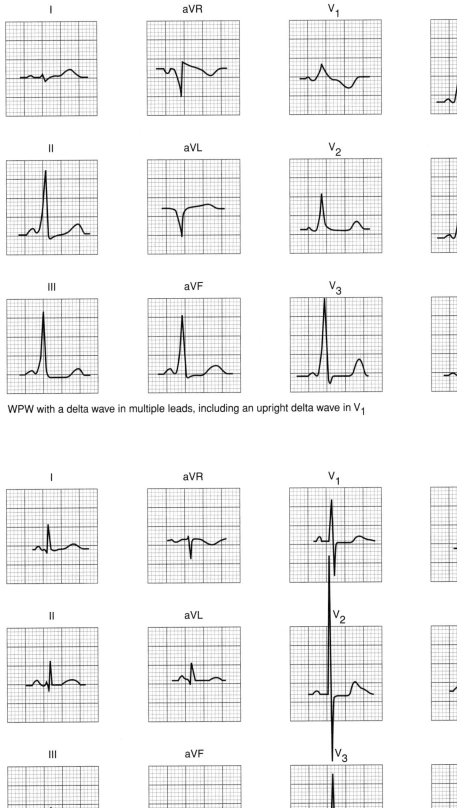

I aVR V₁ V₄

II aVL V₂ V₅

III aVF V₃ V₆

WPW with a delta wave in multiple leads, including an upright delta wave in V₁

I aVR V₁ V₄

II aVL V₂ V₅

III aVF V₃ V₆

Extremely prominent R waves in V₁ and V₂ in a patient with HOCM and asymmetric septal hypertrophy

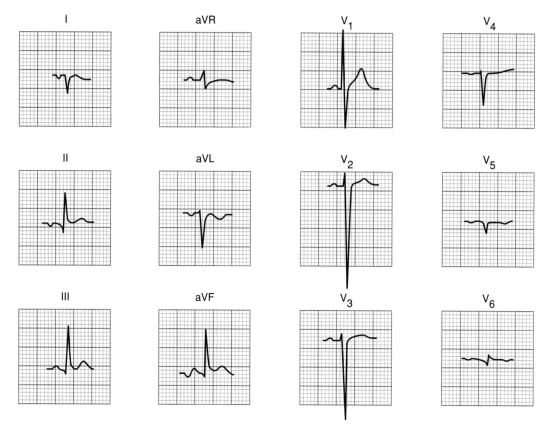

Congenital dextrocardia manifested by right axis deviation, inverted P waves in I and aVF, tall R waves in V_1, and R wave diminution across the precordium

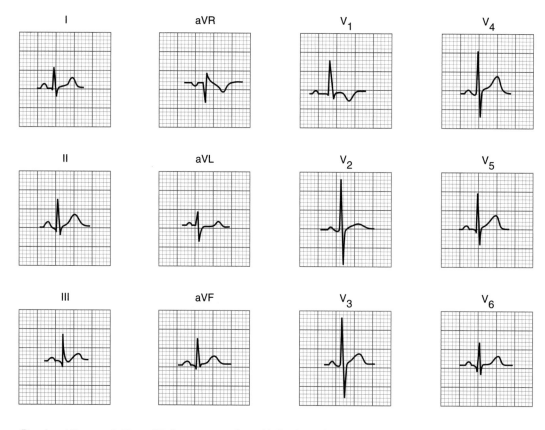

Prominent R waves in V_1 and V_2 in a young patient with Duchenne's muscular dystrophy

V.   Causes of ST segment elevation

   A.   Acute myocardial injury

   B.   Early repolarization

   C.   Acute pericarditis

   D.   LVH

   E.   LBBB

   F.   Hyperkalemia

   G.   Hypothermia

   H.   Scorpion sting

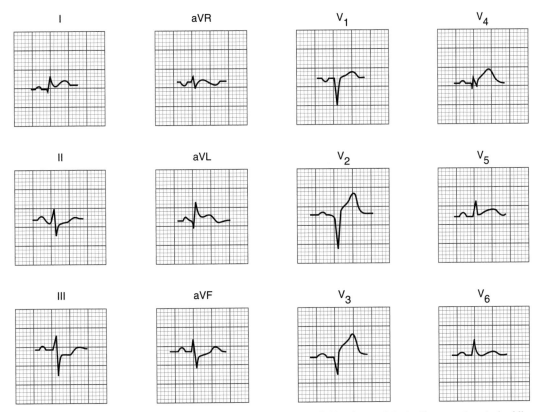

ST segment elevation and Q wave formation in the anterior precordial leads consistent with an acute anterior MI

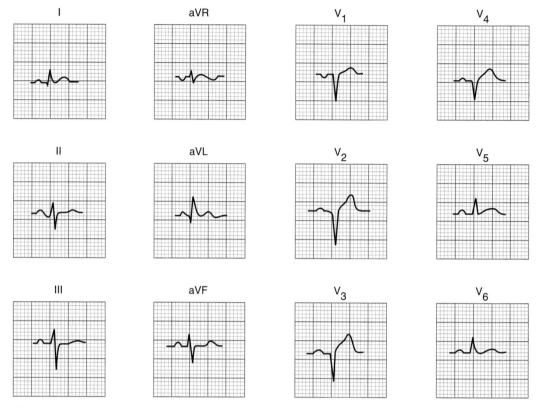

The same patient as above 8 weeks later. There has been resolution of ST depression in the inferior leads, but ST elevation persists in the anterior precordial leads, suggesting the development of a left ventricular aneurysm.

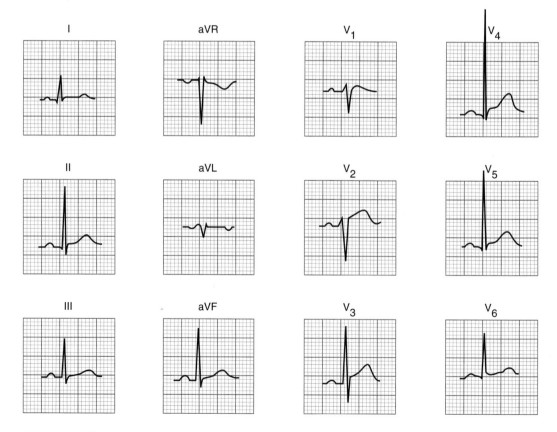

Widespread ST segment elevation in a healthy patient, consistent with early repolarization

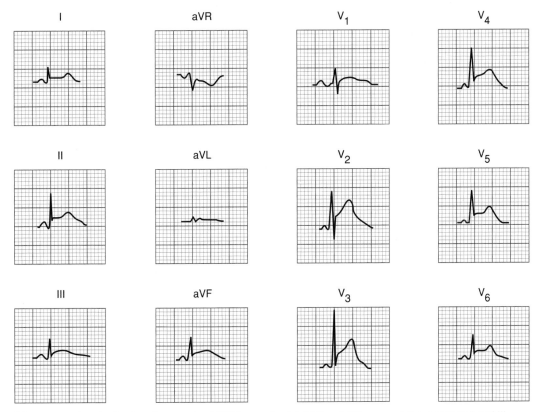

ST segment elevation in virtually every lead (ST depression in aVR) and PR segment depression in II and III, demonstrating acute pericarditis

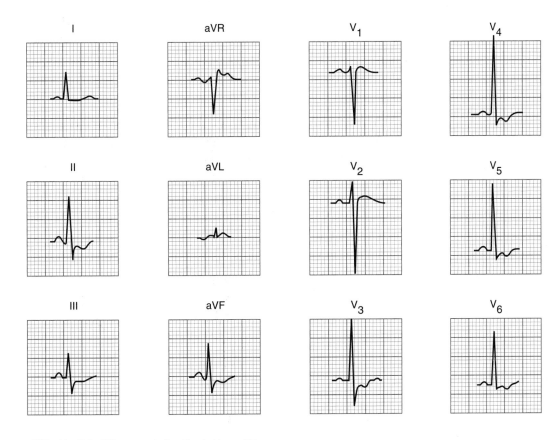

LVH with slight ST segment elevation in V_1 and V_2

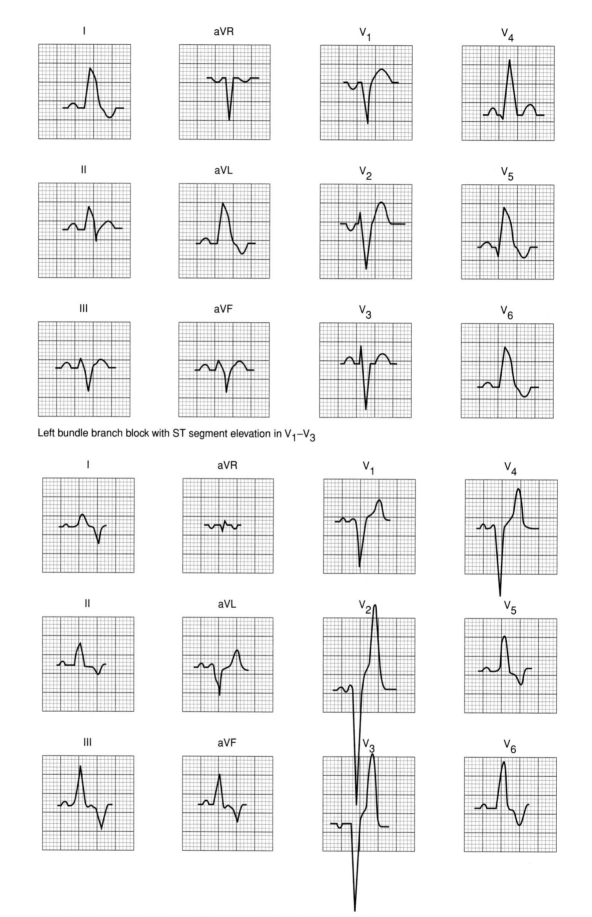

I aVR V$_1$ V$_4$

II aVL V$_2$ V$_5$

III aVF V$_3$ V$_6$

Left bundle branch block with ST segment elevation in V$_1$–V$_3$

I aVR V$_1$ V$_4$

II aVL V$_2$ V$_5$

III aVF V$_3$ V$_6$

Prominent T waves and widespread ST segment elevation in hyperkalemia

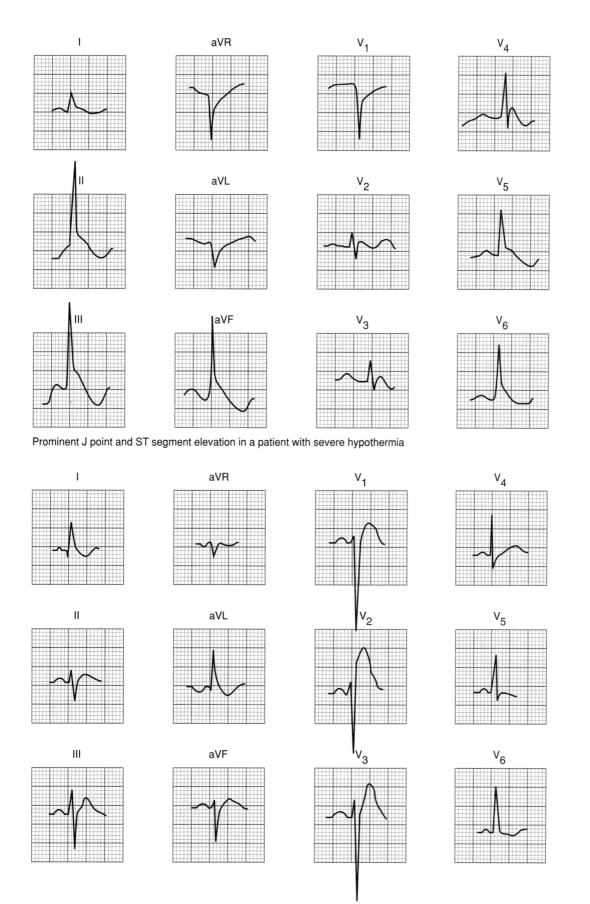

Prominent J point and ST segment elevation in a patient with severe hypothermia

Diffuse ST segment changes in a child stung by an Indian red scorpion [from Bawaskar HS and Bawaskar PH, Management of the cardiovascular manifestations of poisoning by the Indian red scorpion (*Mesobuthus tamulus*). Br Heart J 1992;68:478–480]

VI. CNS injury and the ECG

   A. Severe acute CNS lesions, typically subarachnoid hemorrhage, are
       occasionally associated with ST segment and T wave changes.

   B. The most likely explanation for these changes is unilateral perturbation
       of the sympathetic ganglia at the base of the brain.

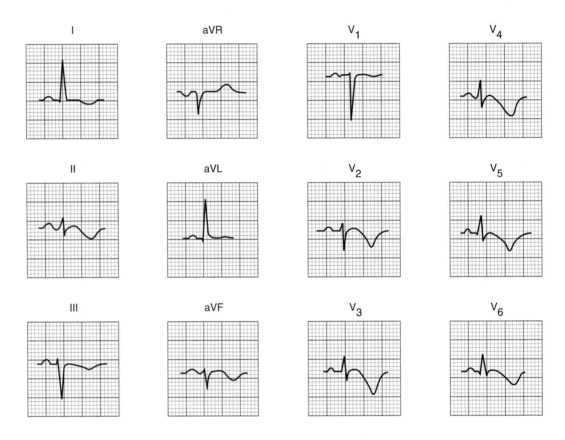

Prominent T wave inversions in a patient with an acute intracerebral hemorrhage

Day 9 ECG 1

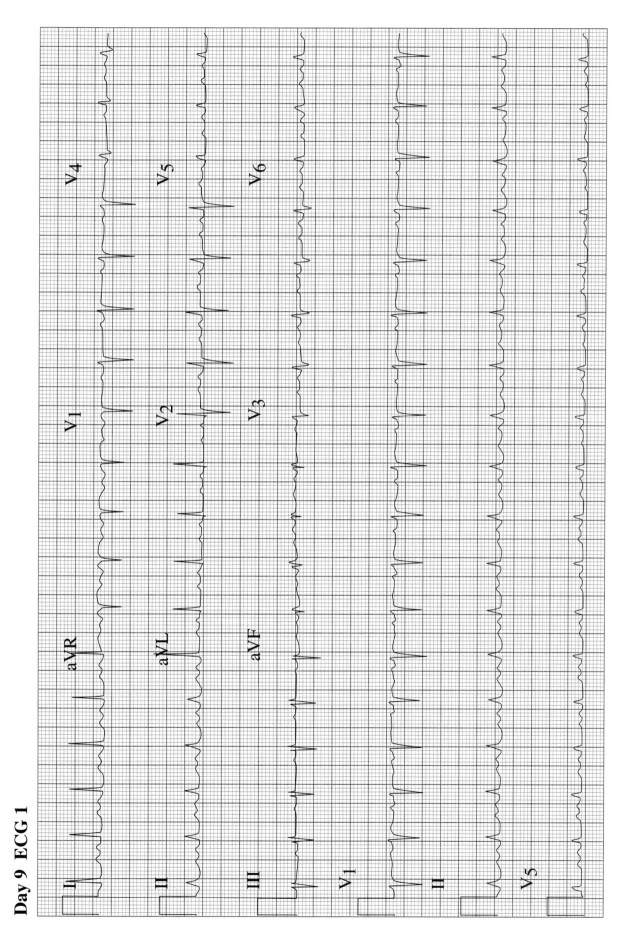

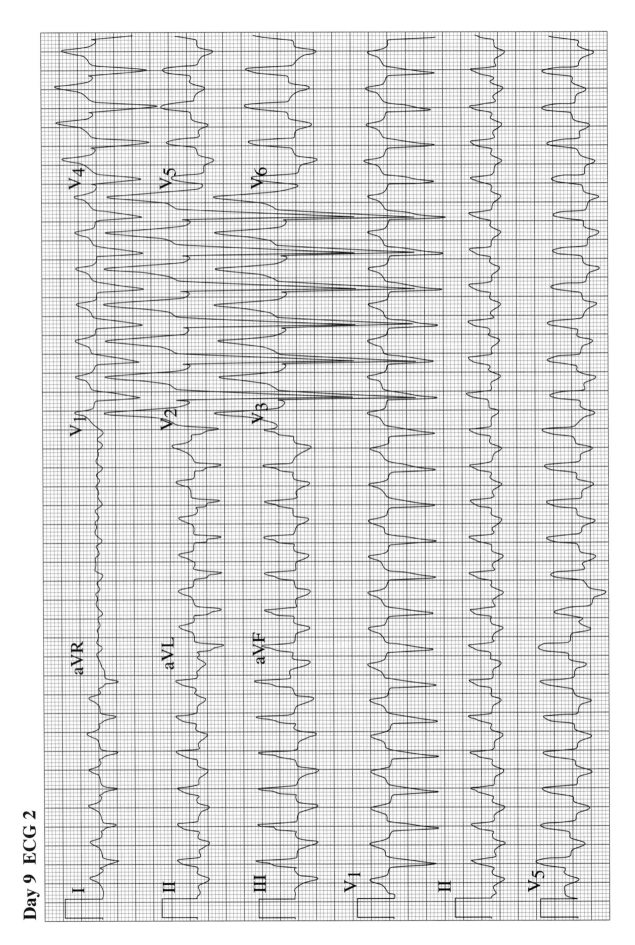

Day 9 ECG 2

Day 9 ECG 3

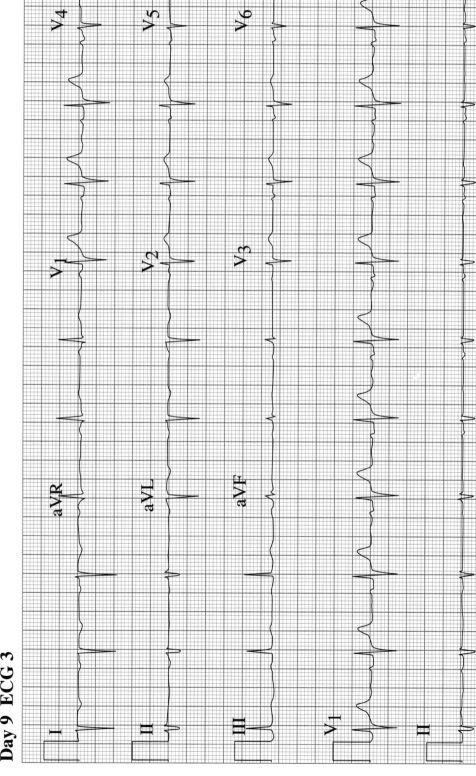

227

Day 9 ECG 4

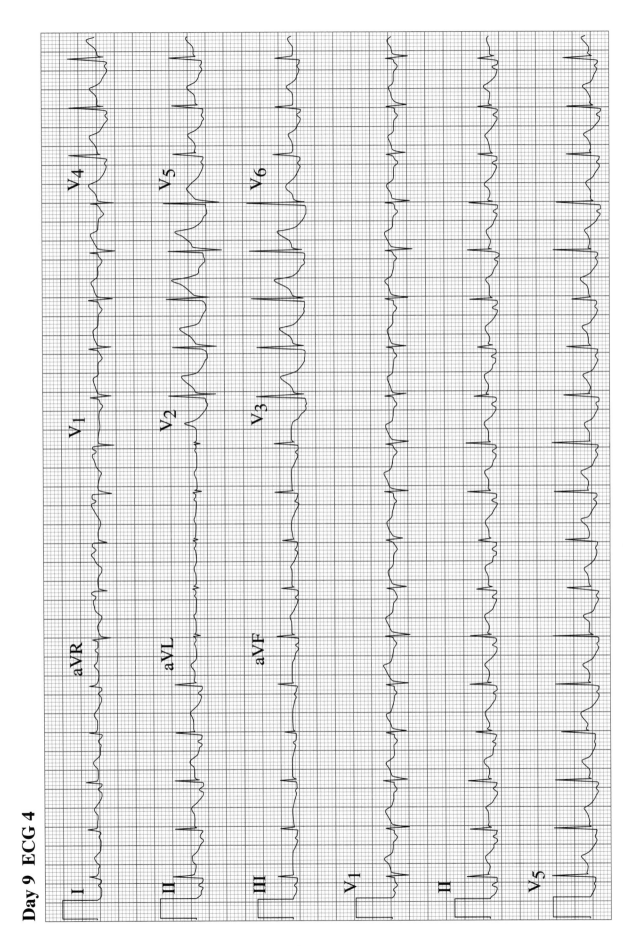

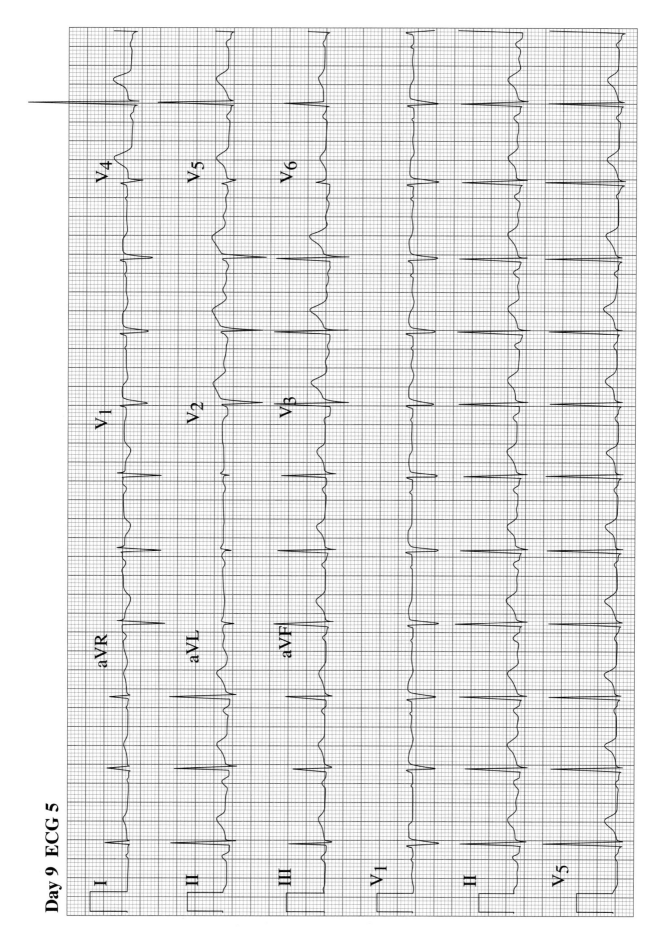

Day 9 ECG 5

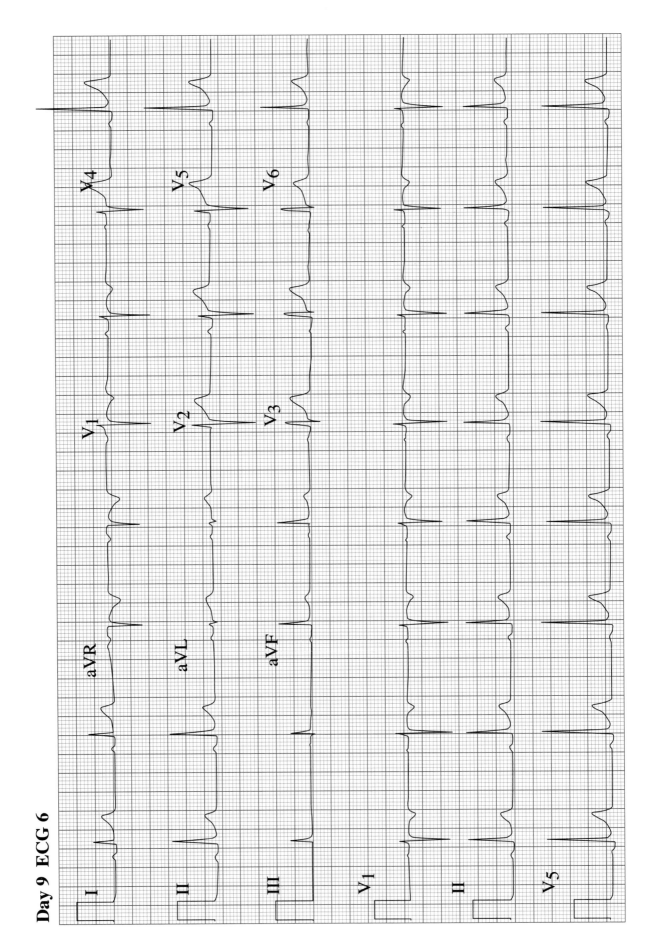

Day 9 ECG 6

230

Day 9 ECG 7

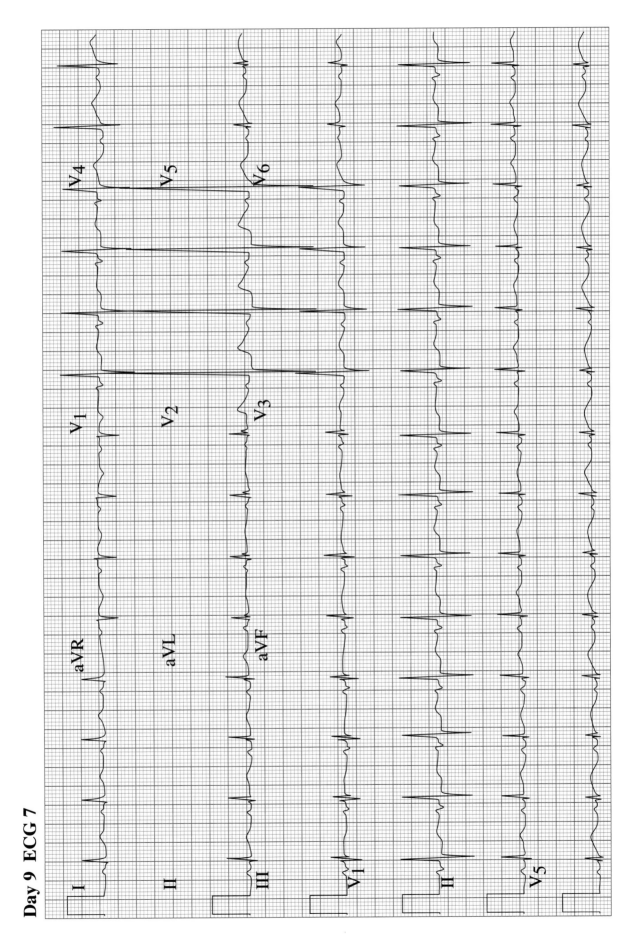

I aVR V₁ V₄

II aVL V₂ V₅

III aVF V₃ V₆

V₁

II

V₅

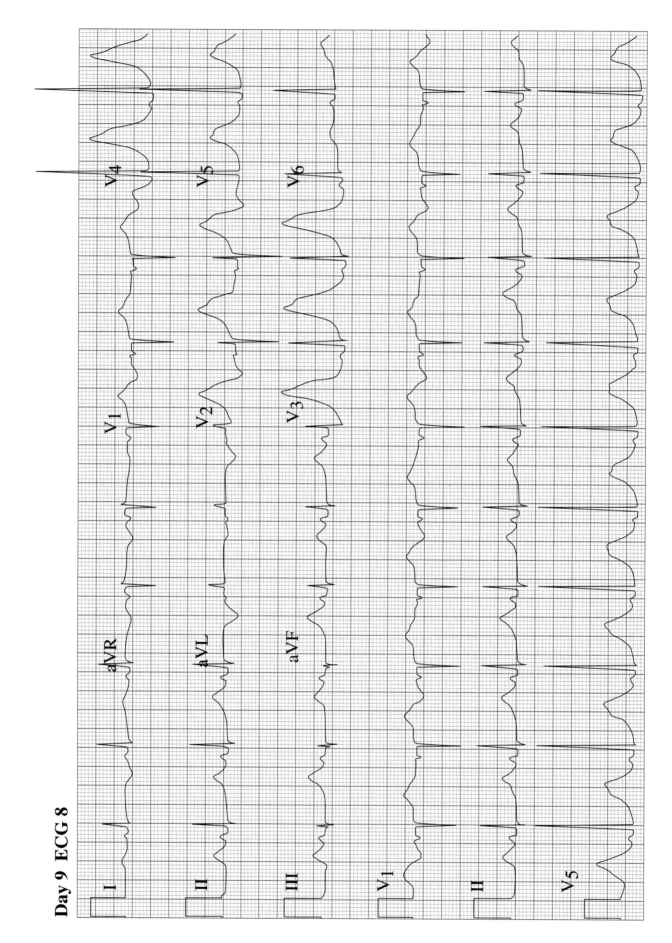

Day 9 ECG 8

I aVR V1 V4

II aVL V2 V5

III aVF V3 V6

V1

II

V5

Day 9 ECG 9

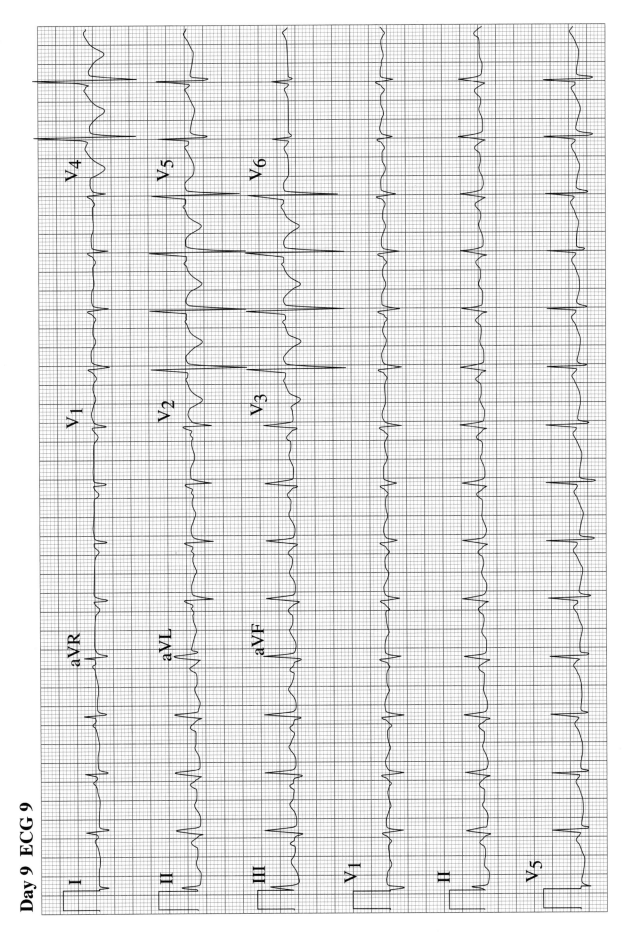

Day 9 ECG 10

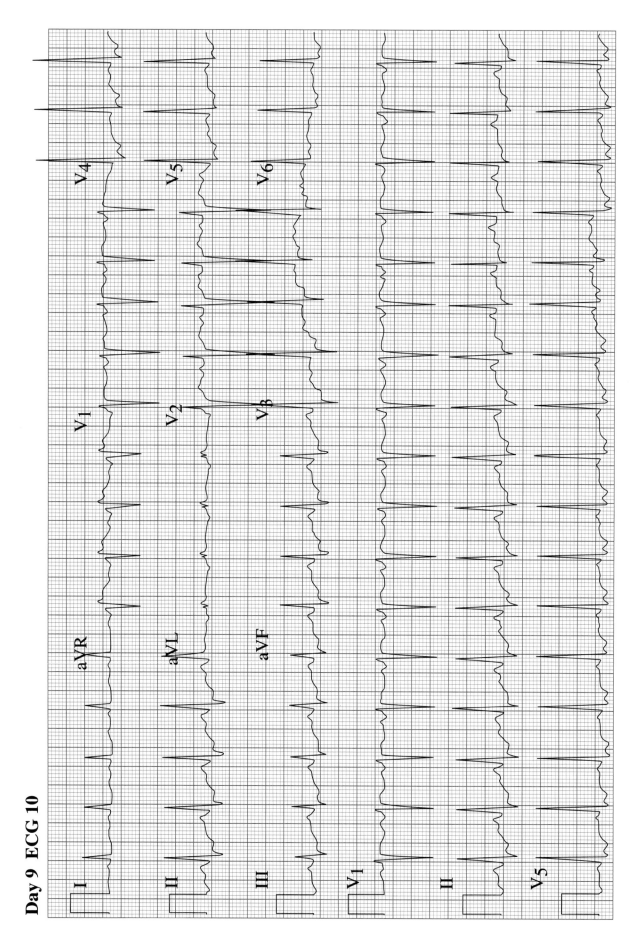

234

Day 9
ECG Interpretations and Discussion

Day 9 ECG 1
Sinus tachycardia
Long QT interval

This long QT interval has a unique morphology. The shape of the T wave is normal but the ST segment is greatly prolonged. This is highly suggestive of hypocalcemia, which was confirmed clinically.

Day 9 ECG 2
Sinus tachycardia
Nonspecific intraventricular conduction defect
Peaked T waves

These bizarre-appearing QRS complexes demonstrate extremely peaked T waves. This patient had a potassium level of 7.0 mg/dL.

Day 9 ECG 3
Normal sinus rhythm
Congenital dextrocardia

The P wave and the QRS axis are rightward, there is a tall R wave in V_1, and there are diminishing R waves across the precordium. This ECG is typical of *situs inversus* dextrocardia. Reversing all of the ECG leads would result in a normal tracing.

Day 9 ECG 4
Sinus tachycardia
Acute pericarditis

There is ST segment elevation in all the leads except aVR, in which there is ST depression. There is also PR segment depression in several leads, most obviously in II.

Day 9 ECG 5
Normal sinus rhythm
Left ventricular hypertrophy with repolarization abnormalities

The ST segment elevation in this patient is associated with left ventricular hypertrophy.

Day 9 ECG 6

    Sinus bradycardia

    Early repolarization

There is ST segment elevation in several leads with no other obvious cause than early repolarization. This ECG is from a young healthy African American male in whom these findings are common.

Day 9 ECG 7

    Normal sinus rhythm

    Nonspecific ST and T wave changes

    Long QT interval

There are extremely prominent R waves in V_1 and V_2 due to asymmetric septal hypertrophy associated with hypertrophic cardiomyopathy. These findings were demonstrated on echocardiography.

Day 9 ECG 8

    Normal sinus rhythm

    Nonspecific ST changes

    Prominent T waves in the precordial leads

    Prolonged QT interval

This patient had an episode of prolonged severe ischemia when this ECG was obtained.

Day 9 ECG 9

    Normal sinus rhythm

    Probable inferior MI, age undetermined

    Diffuse T wave inversion

This patient presented with an acute neurological deficit and had a subarachnoid hemorrhage on CT scan.

Day 9 ECG 10

    Sinus tachycardia

    Nonspecific ST and T wave abnormalities

This 32-year-old female had a tricyclic antidepressant overdose.

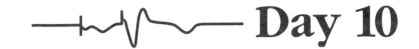 **Day 10**

Electronic Pacemakers

I.   Pacemaker nomenclature

    A.   A standardized letter code has been designated for the various pacemaker functions.

    B.   The first letter (P) of the code indicates the chamber(s) paced.

    C.   The second letter (S) indicates the chamber(s) sensed.

    D.   The third letter (A) indicates the pacemaker activity—triggered, inhibited, or neither.

    E.   The fourth letter (R) indicates the presence or absence of rate responsiveness.

    F.   The fifth letter relates to antitachycardia functions, advanced features which are beyond the scope of this text.

II. Pacemaker development

    A.   VOO
        1.   The first pacemakers, developed in the late 1950s, had no sensing circuitry and paced in the ventricle at a rate set at the factory.
        2.   The advantage of this system was that it was better than asystole.

P	S	A
Chamber Paced	Chamber Sensed	Activity
V	O	O

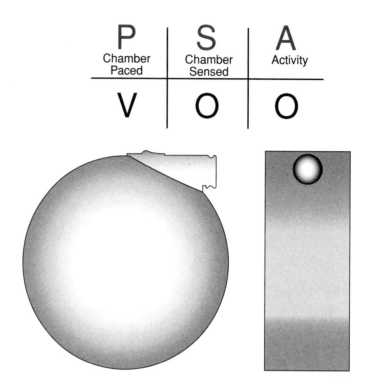

First generation pacemaker— paces in the ventricle, does not sense, and is neither triggered nor inhibited. The pacemaker is portrayed actual size from the front and side

Problems associated with VOO mode:

A. "R on T" phenomenon
B. Uses battery constantly
C. Distorts all QRS complexes
D. No AV synchrony
E. No rate responsiveness

Lead II—sinus rhythm, third degree AV block, and a VOO pacemaker. Note the AV dissociation. The premature junctional beat (arrow) is not sensed by the pacemaker and does not change the pacemaker timing.

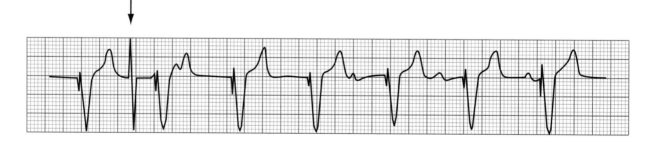

B. VVT
   1. This pacemaker sensed in the ventricle, but was committed to firing.
   2. This technology solved the potential problem of ventricular arrhythmia genesis by avoiding firing on the upslope of the T wave.

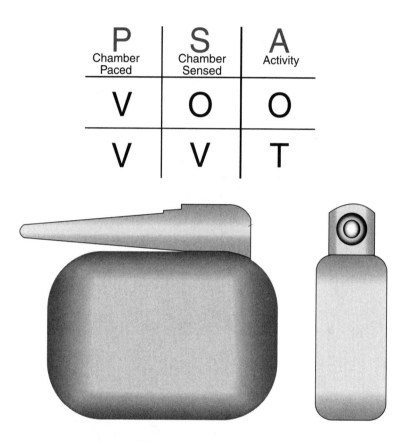

P Chamber Paced	**S** Chamber Sensed	**A** Activity
V	O	O
V	V	T

Second generation pacemaker— paces in the ventricle, senses in the ventricle, and is triggered. Pacemaker is portrayed actual size from the front and side

Problems associated with VVT mode:

A.   ~~"R on T" phenomenon~~
B.   Uses battery constantly
C.   Distorts all QRS complexes
D.   No AV synchrony
E.   No rate responsiveness

Lead II—junctional rhythm and a VVT pacemaker. The premature junctional beat (arrow) is sensed by the pacemaker, and the pacemaker discharges on top of the premature beat. The interval following the premature beat is a typical pacing interval.

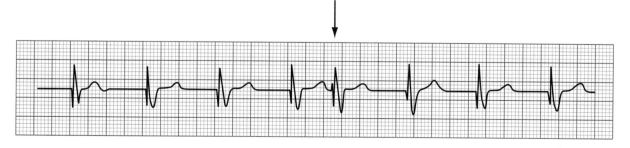

C. VVI
  1. This pacemaker sensed in the ventricle and fired only if a ventricular beat did not occur during the programmed timing cycle.
  2. This technology decreased battery utilization and deformation of every QRS complex.

P Chamber Paced	S Chamber Sensed	A Activity
V	O	O
V	V	T
V	V	I

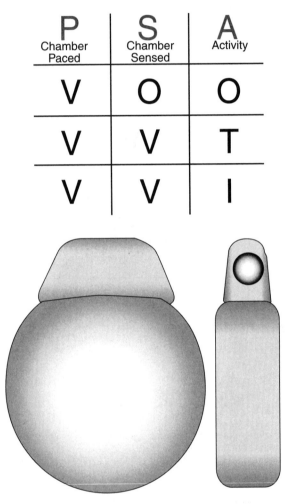

Third generation pacemaker— paces in the ventricle, senses in the ventricle, and is inhibited. The basic rate is programmable. Pacemaker is portrayed actual size from the front and side.

Problems associated with VVT mode:

A. ~~"R on T" phenomenon~~
B. ~~Uses battery constantly~~
C. ~~Distorts all QRS complexes~~
D. No AV synchrony
E. No rate responsiveness

Lead II—sinus rhythm, third degree AV block, and a VVI pacemaker. A premature junctional beat (arrow) is sensed by the pacemaker, and the pacemaker is inhibited. The interval following the premature beat is a typical pacing interval.

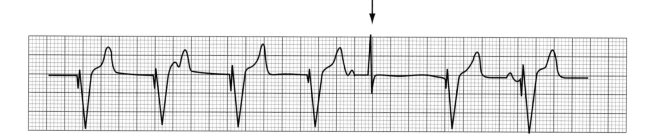

D. AV sequential pacemakers
   1. AV sequential pacemakers, often referred to by the code DDD (for Dual, Dual, Dual), pace and sense in the atrium and the ventricle, and can be inhibited or triggered.

P Chamber Paced	S Chamber Sensed	A Activity
V	O	O
V	V	T
V	V	I
D	D	D

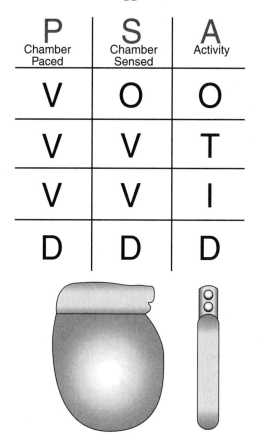

Fourth generation pacemaker— paces in the atrium and ventricle, senses in the atrium and ventricle, and can be programmed to be inhibited or triggered. DDD stands for Dual, Dual, Dual. The ventricular rate and the AV delay are programmable. Pacemaker is portrayed actual size from the front and side.

Problems associated with DDD mode:

A. ~~"R on T" phenomenon~~
B. ~~Uses battery constantly~~
C. ~~Distorts all QRS complexes~~
D. ~~No AV synchrony~~
E. No rate responsiveness

2. The typical setting for these units is DDI, in which the pacing functions are inhibited by appropriate atrial and ventricular depolarization.
3. There are two basic intervals which must be programmed:
    a. The V-V interval—this is the time between ventricular depolarizations, or the basic heart rate.
    b. The A-V delay—this is the time between atrial and ventricular depolarization.
4. With the V-V interval and A-V delay programmed, there are four possible responses by the pacemaker.
5. AV sequential pacemakers allow AV synchrony, which may substantially improve stroke volume.

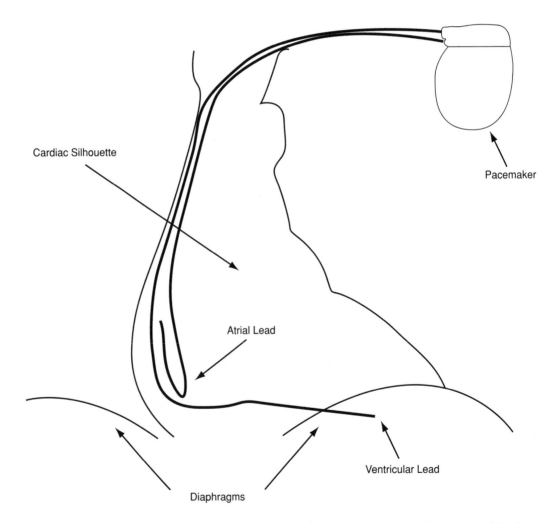

Outline of a chest X-ray showing the location of a DDD pacemaker and the atrial and ventricular leads. Note the atrial lead curled in the right atrium and lodged in the atrial appendage. The ventricular lead is in the RV apex.

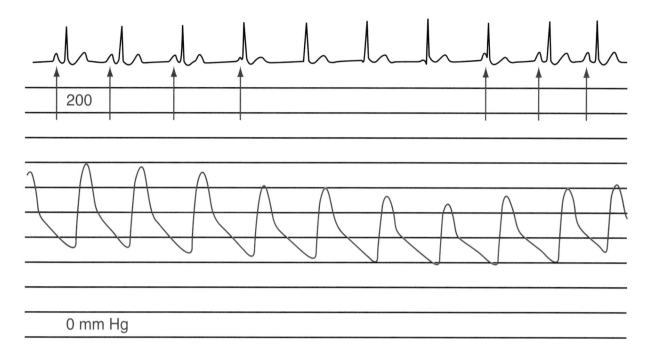

Simultaneous Lead II rhythm strip and arterial pressure in a patient undergoing cardiac catheterization. In the center of the strip, he spontaneously developed sinus bradycardia with a junctional escape rhythm (P waves are indicated by the red arrows). The temporary loss of AV synchrony produced a substantial fall in arterial blood pressure.

E. Rate responsive pacemakers
1. These devices have the ability to detect increasing patient activity, usually by sensing pectoral muscle artifact.
2. The heart rate is increased according to programmed parameters.
3. After exercise ceases, the heart rate slows down gradually, again according to programmed parameters.
4. Both VVI and DDD pacemakers can utilize this technology.

Response 1—the patient's own QRS starts the V-V clock. The pacemaker knows that a P wave must occur within 800 msec (1000 minus 200). In this case, a native P wave occurs within 800 msec and the A-V clock starts. The native P wave inhibits the atrial pacemaker, so no atrial spike is seen. The patient has his own ventricular depolarization within 200 msec which inhibits the ventricular pacemaker. No ventricular spike is seen.

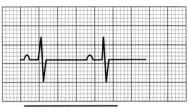

1000 msec

Response 2—in this case, a P wave does not occur within 800 msec, so the atrial pacemaker discharges and produces an odd-axis P wave. The A-V clock starts, the patient has his own ventricular depolarization within 200 msec and inhibits the ventricular pacemaker. No ventricular spike is seen.

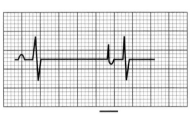

200 msec

Response 3—in this case, a P wave does occur within 800 msec, so the atrial pacemaker is inhibited. The A-V clock starts, but there is no native ventricular depolarization within 200 msec and the ventricular pacemaker discharges, producing a wide QRS complex.

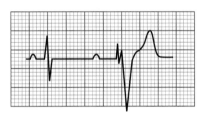

Response 4—in this case, a P wave does not occur within 800 msec, so the atrial pacemaker discharges and produces an odd-axis P wave. The A-V clock starts, but there is no native ventricular depolarization within 200 msec and the ventricular pacemaker discharges, producing a wide QRS complex.

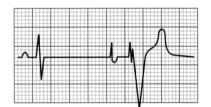

The 4 types of response by an AV sequential pacemaker programmed with a V-V interval of 1000 msec (1 sec; heart rate of 60) and an A-V delay of 200 msec.

Lead II—a paced rhythm with a VVI pacemaker. Note the retrograde P waves following each paced beat. This patient would benefit from an AV sequential pacemaker.

Lead II—sinus rhythm with third degree AV block and a VVI pacemaker. This patient would benefit from an AV sequential pacemaker.

Lead II—sinus bradycardia with an AV sequential pacemaker. The pacemaker is tracking the atrium and discharging in the ventricle.

Lead II—AV sequential pacing with both the atrial and ventricular pacemakers discharging.

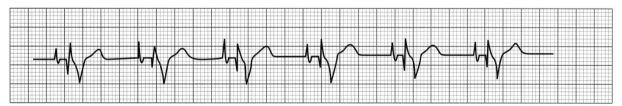

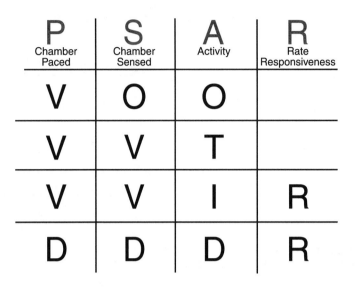

P Chamber Paced	S Chamber Sensed	A Activity	R Rate Responsiveness
V	O	O	
V	V	T	
V	V	I	R
D	D	D	R

Fifth generation pacemakers—these devices have the ability to detect increasing physical activity by the patient, usually by sensing pectoral muscle artifact. These pacemakers can increase the heart rate according to programmed parameters. Both VVI and DDD pacemakers can utilize this technology.

Problems solved by DDDR mode:

A.   ~~"R on T" phenomenon~~
B.   ~~Uses battery constantly~~
C.   ~~Distorts all QRS complexes~~
D.   ~~No AV synchrony~~
E.   ~~No rate responsiveness~~

Lead II—a paced rhythm with a VVI pacemaker. There are tiny retrograde P waves following each paced beat. This patient would benefit from an AV sequential pacemaker.

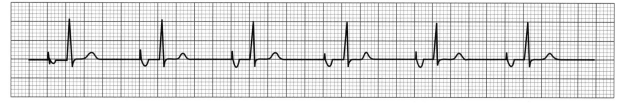

Lead II—AV sequential pacemaker with atrial pacing, normal AV conduction, and appropriate inhibition of the ventricular pacemaker

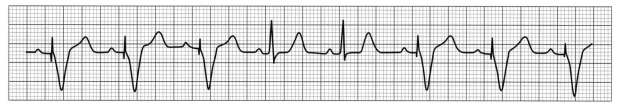

Lead II—sinus rhythm and AV sequential pacing. Note the two beats in the center which have normal AV conduction, thus inhibiting the ventricular pacemaker.

Lead II—atrial fibrillation and a VVI pacemaker pacing the ventricle. This is a rate responsive pacemaker (VVIR), and will respond to physical activity.

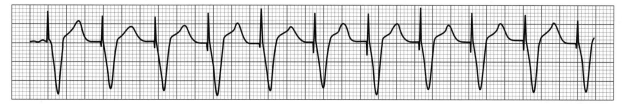

Lead II—the same patient as above during physical activity. The VVIR pacemaker has increased the heart rate appropriately.

III. Technical problems with pacemakers

    A. "R on T" phenomenon
        1. There was a great deal of concern that a pacemaker without sensing capabilities could discharge on the upslope of the T wave.
        2. There was concern that this situation could initiate VT or VF.

    B. Constant battery drain
        1. Early pacemakers used zinc oxide batteries which limited the pacemaker to about 1 year of operation.
        2. Advances in battery technology have extended the life expectancy of modern pacemakers to 7 years or more.

    C. The pacemaker distorted all QRS complexes, making other ECG diagnoses difficult or impossible.

    D. There was no atrioventricular synchrony.

    E. There was no rate responsiveness.

    F. These problems have been solved by advanced technology.

IV. Pacemaker leads

    A. Unipolar leads
        1. Unipolar leads have one electrode at the tip, and the pacemaker box serves as the other electrode.
        2. The pacemaker spikes are very tall and obvious.

    B. Bipolar leads
        1. Bipolar leads have one electrode at the tip of the lead and another about 1 cm proximally.
        2. Bipolar leads produce tiny spikes on the ECG which are easily overlooked.

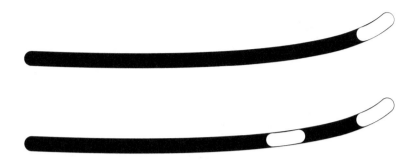

The distal ends of a unipolar (upper) and a bipolar (lower) pacemaker lead

Lead II—atrial fibrillation and a VVI pacemaker pacing the ventricle. The narrow complex in the center occurs before the programmed ventricular interval and inhibits the pacemaker. The lead, as evidenced by the very large pacing spikes, is unipolar.

Lead II—sinus rhythm, third degree AV block, and a VVI pacemaker. The lead, as evidenced by the tiny pacing spikes, is bipolar.

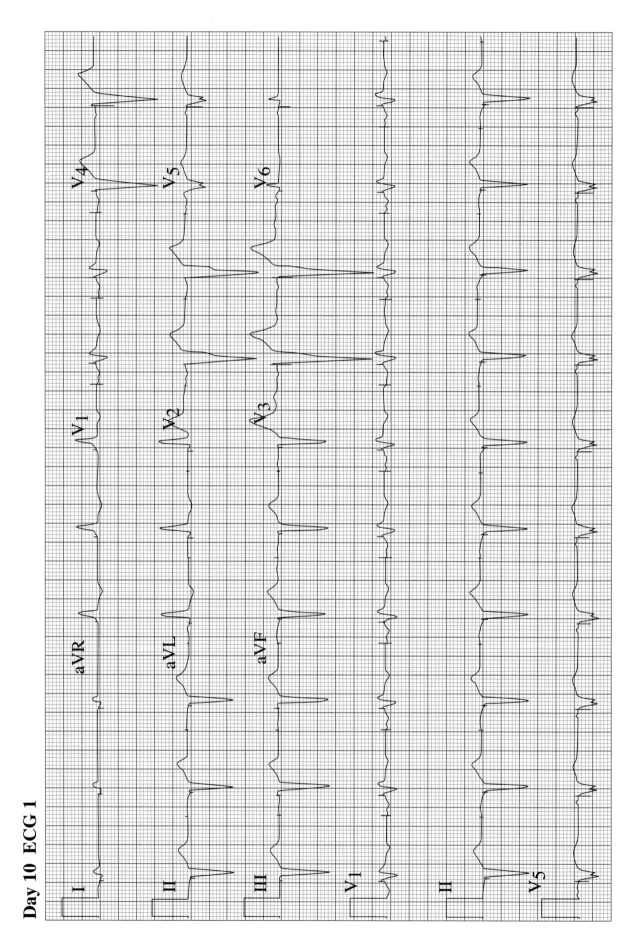

Day 10 ECG 2

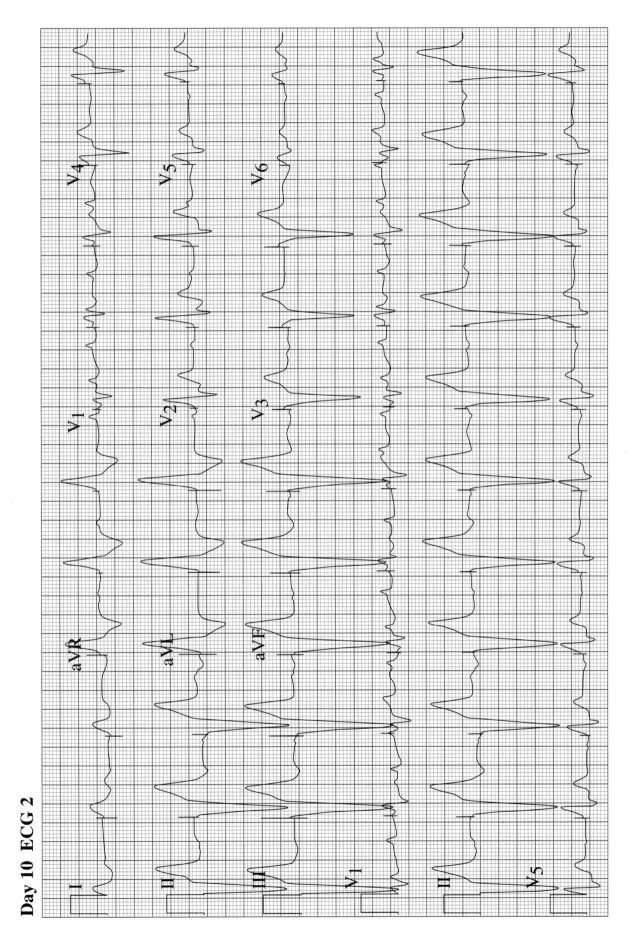

Day 10 ECG 3

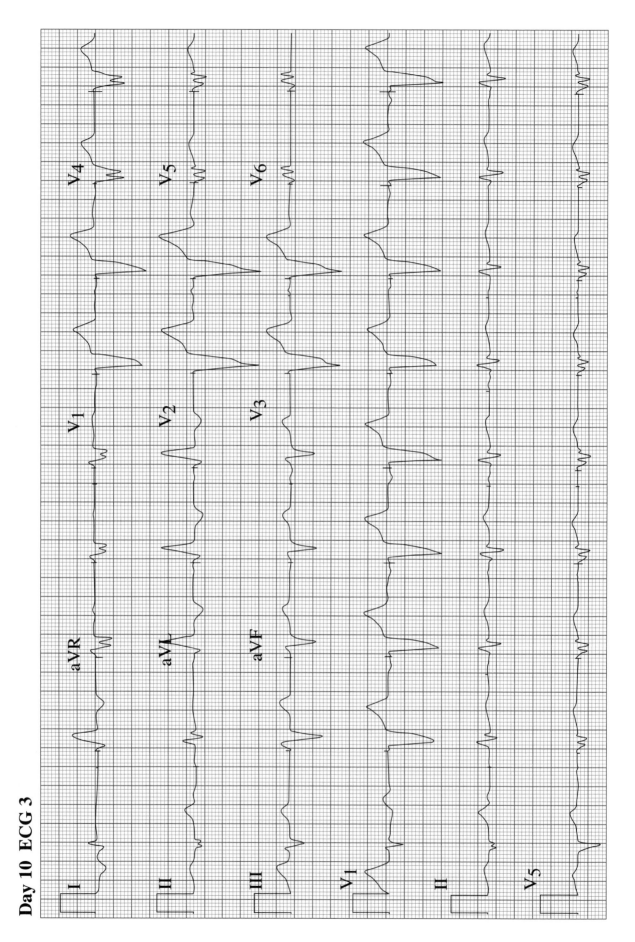

252

Day 10 ECG 4

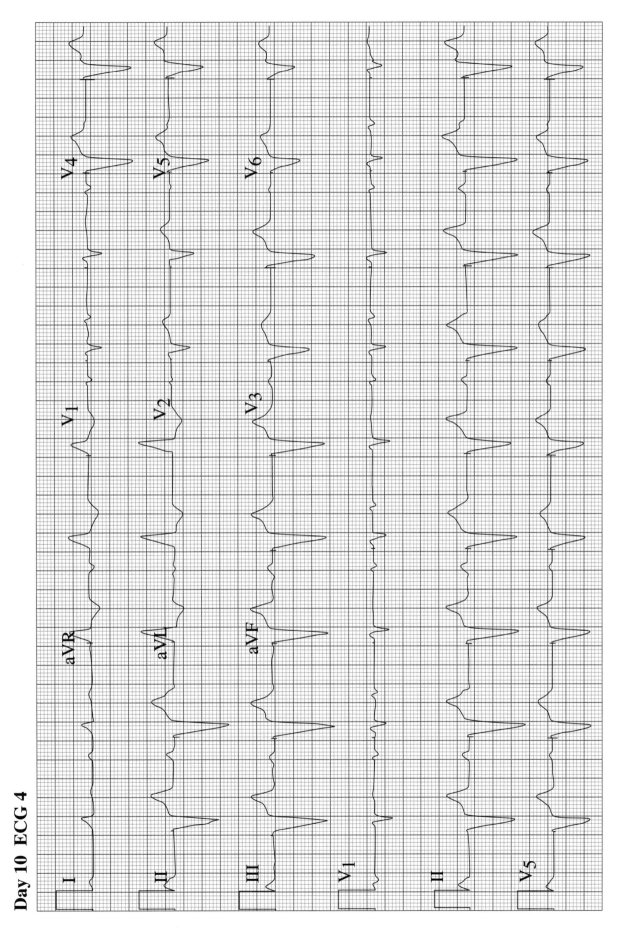

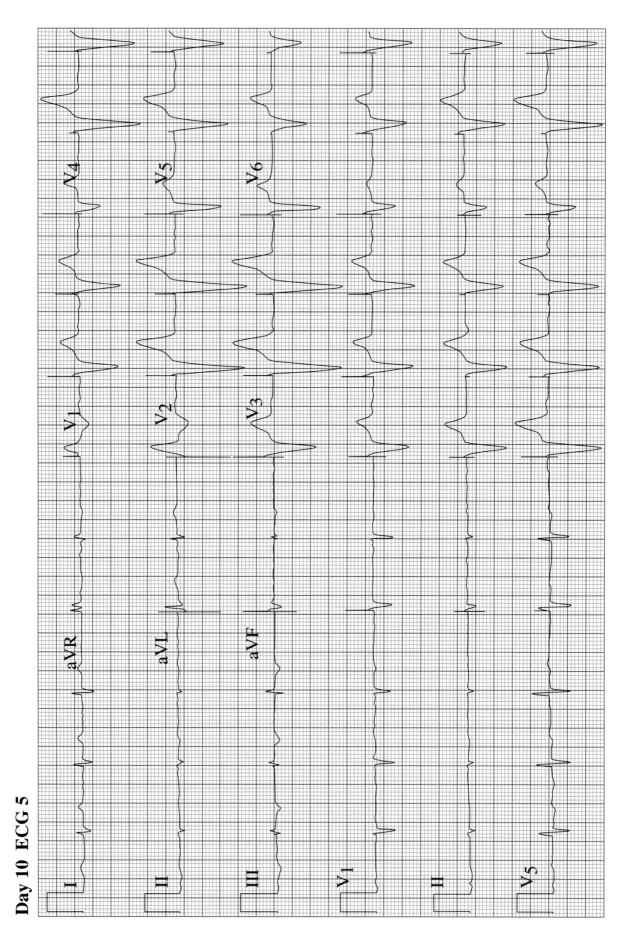

Day 10 ECG 5

Day 10 ECG 6

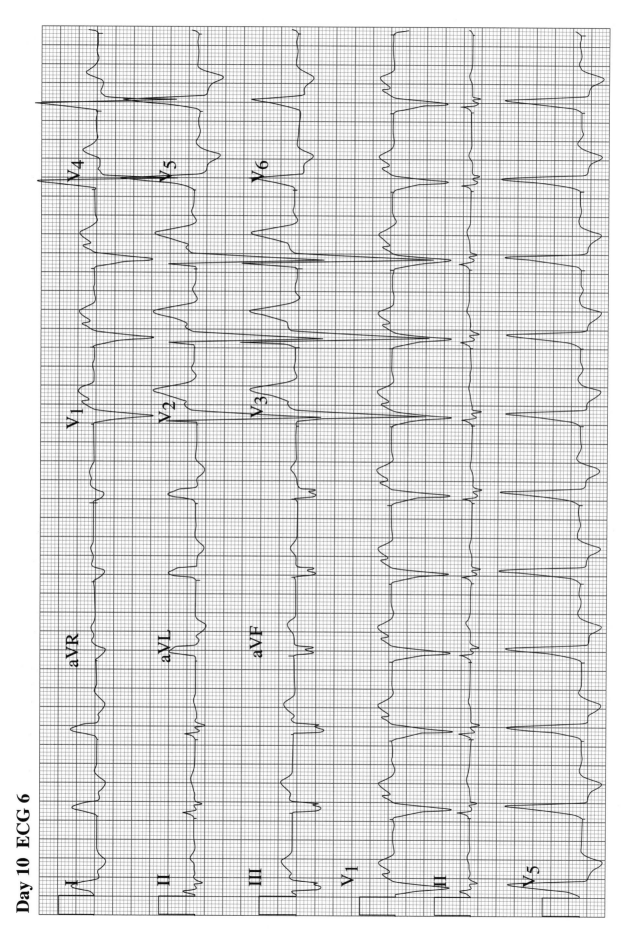

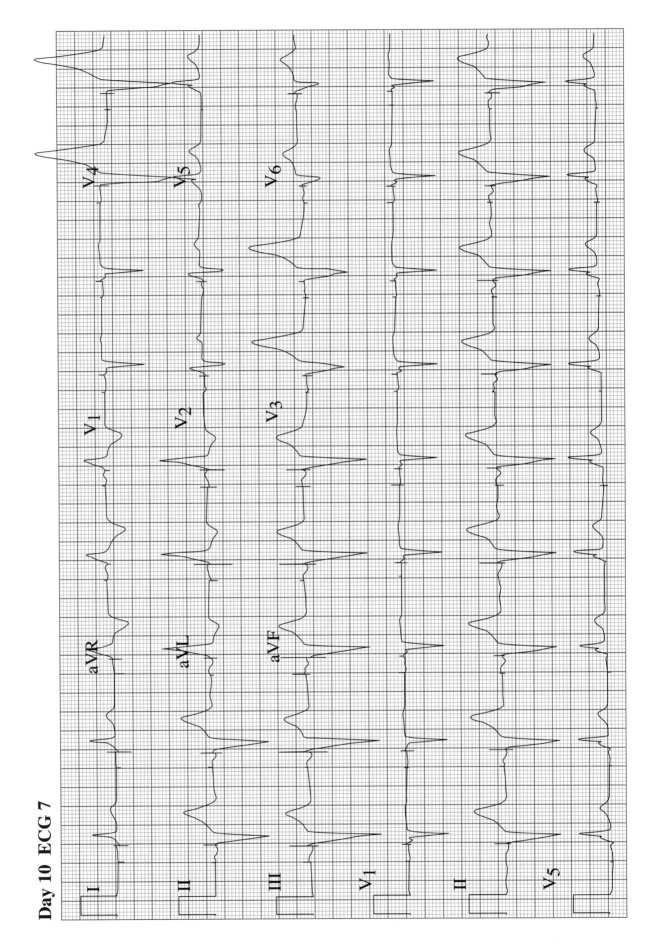

Day 10 ECG 7

I   aVR   V1   V4

II   aVL   V2   V5

III   aVF   V3   V6

V1

II

V5

Day 10 ECG 8

** All leads at half standard**

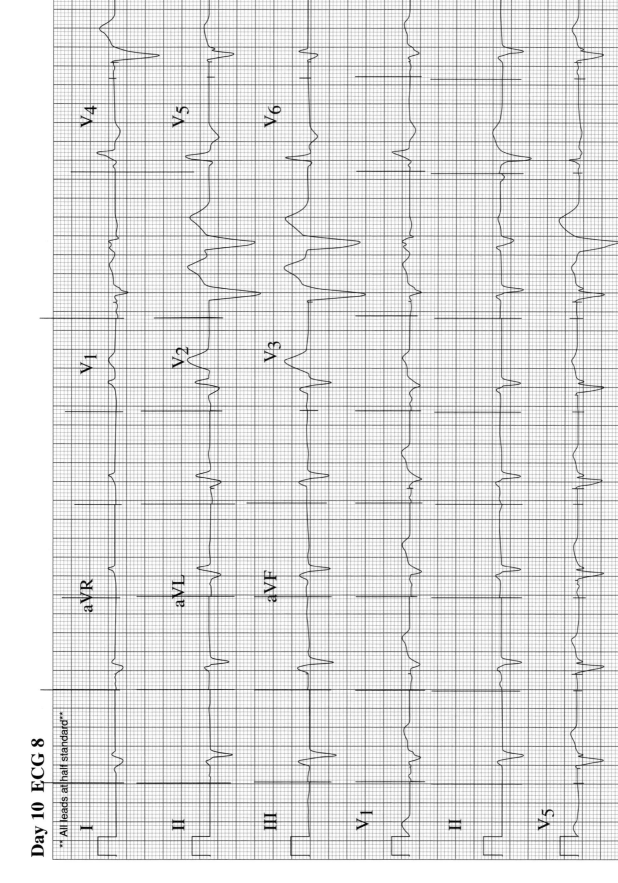

I   aVR   V₁   V₄

II   aVL   V₂   V₅

III   aVF   V₃   V₆

V₁

II

V₅

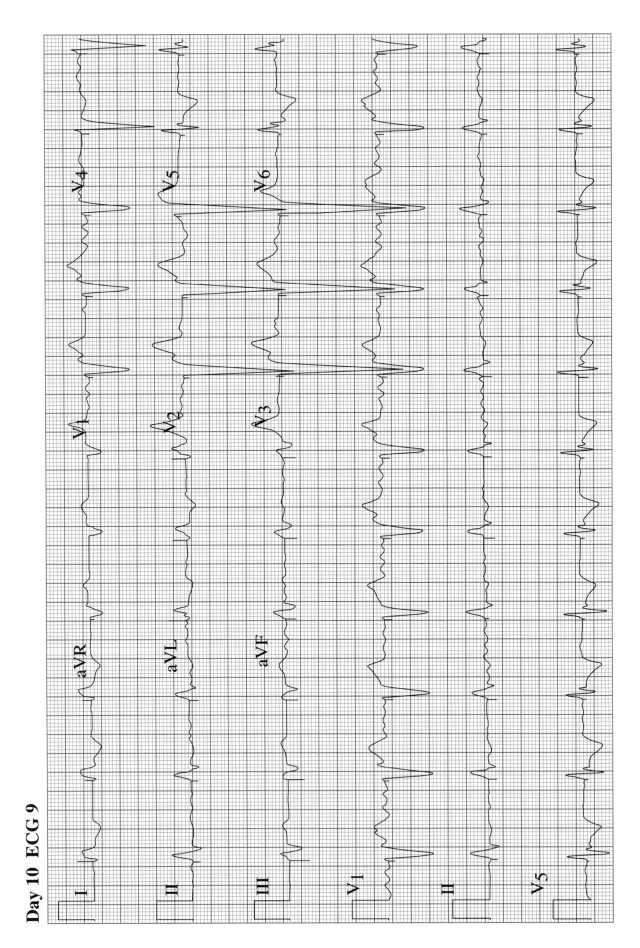

Day 10 ECG 9

I

II

III

V1

II

V5

aVR

aVL

aVF

V1

V2

V3

V4

V5

V6

Day 10 ECG 10

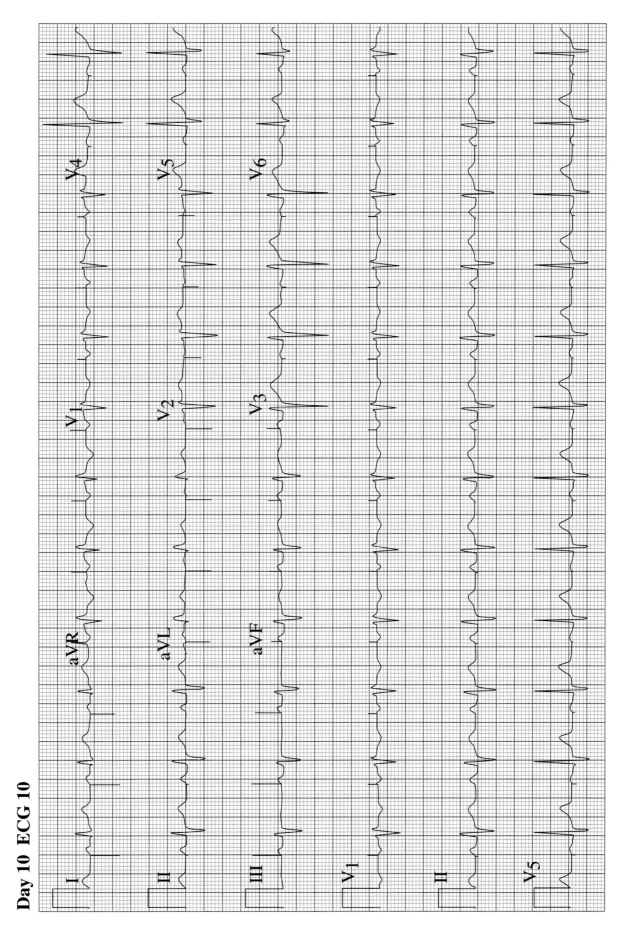

Day 10
ECG Interpretations and Discussion

Day 10 ECG 1
   Electronic pacemaker with atrial and ventricular pacing

There are pacemaker spikes prior to atrial and ventricular depolarizations.

Day 10 ECG 2
   Electronic pacemaker with ventricular pacing
   Underlying rhythm is atrial tachycardia
   Third degree AV block

There is an underlying fairly rapid supraventricular rhythm with an unusual P wave axis indicating atrial tachycardia. None of these impulses are conducted to the ventricle, consistent with third degree AV block. There is a ventricular pacemaker.

Day 10 ECG 3
   Electronic pacemaker with atrial and ventricular pacing
   Left axis deviation
   Inferior MI, age undetermined

The left axis deviation and the inferior MI are only apparent in the first non-paced QRS complex.

Day 10 ECG 4
   Electronic pacemaker with ventricular pacing
   Underlying rhythm is sinus
   Third degree AV block

This patient might benefit from a pacemaker with both atrial and ventricular pacing capabilities.

Day 10 ECG 5
   Atrial fibrillation and an electronic pacemaker with ventricular pacing
   Possible inferior MI, age undetermined

This pacemaker is functioning in the VVI mode, in that the pacemaker is inhibited at the beginning of the tracing.

Day 10 ECG 6
   Electronic ventricular pacemaker with ventricular pacing
   Retrograde atrial activation

This patient might benefit from a pacemaker with both atrial and ventricular pacing capabilities.

Day 10 ECG 7
   Electronic pacemaker with atrial and ventricular pacing

Day 10 ECG 8
   Ventricular pacemaker with atrial and ventricular pacing
   Frequent and successive ventricular extrasystoles

The large atrial pacing spikes are indicative of a unipolar lead.

Day 10 ECG 9
   Electronic pacemaker with ventricular pacing
   Underlying rhythm is atrial fibrillation

Atrial pacing would be ineffective in this patient with atrial fibrillation.

Day 10 ECG 10
   Electronic pacemaker with atrial pacing
   Left axis deviation

In this patient, the PR interval is short enough so that ventricular pacing is inhibited.

ECG Course
Final Examination

Please circle all of the correct responses. One or more may be correct:

1. Correct statements regarding electrocardiographic (ECG) intervals include:
   A. The normal PR interval is 120–240 ms.
   B. A QRS duration of $>$ 120 ms is always abnormal.
   C. Digoxin prolongs the QT interval.
   D. Quinidine prolongs the QT interval.
   E. Hypocalcemia prolongs the QT interval.

2. Which of the following statements is/are true regarding third degree AV block?
   A. There is frequently group beating of the QRS complexes.
   B. The atrial rate is always faster than the ventricular rate.
   C. A narrow complex escape rhythm indicates a ventricular focus.
   D. There may be a slight variation in the P-P interval.
   E. Third degree block usually represents a failure of AV nodal, rather than His bundle, conduction.

3. Which of the following statements is/are true regarding intraventricular conduction defects:
   A. An old myocardial infarction (MI) can be read in an ECG with RBBB.
   B. In LBBB, there is a delay in the intrinsicoid deflection time in V_1.
   C. Left anterior fascicular block (LAFB) requires a left axis deviation of $>$ 60°.
   D. In LBBB, there is a monophasic R wave in V_6.
   E. Small Q waves are usually present in I and aVL in LAFB.

4. True statements concerning atrial abnormalities include:
   A. Left or right atrial abnormality can be interpreted from an ECG showing ectopic atrial rhythm.
   B. Peaked P waves in V_1 are indicative of right atrial abnormality.
   C. Notched P waves with a duration of $>$ 120 ms in II, III, and aVF are consistent with left atrial abnormality.
   D. Left atrial abnormality is indicated by a terminal negative portion of the P wave in V_1 which is at least 1 mm deep and 40 ms long.
   E. Simultaneous biatrial abnormalities cannot be interpreted on an ECG.

5. True statements concerning voltage abnormalities of the QRS complex include:
    A. An absolute value of < 10 mm of any limb leads is reported as low voltage.
    B. Myocardial infarction is a frequent cause of low voltage.
    C. An R wave > 13 mm in aVL is consistent with LVH.
    D. A sum of the S wave in V_1 and the R wave in $V_5 > 35$ indicates LVH.
    E. The diagnosis of RVH always requires a tall R wave in V_1.

6. Causes of ST segment elevation include:
    A. Early repolarization
    B. Rattlesnake bite
    C. Digitalis toxicity
    D. Pericarditis
    E. Hypothermia

7. Conditions which may simulate an MI on the ECG include:
    A. LBBB
    B. WPW
    C. Chronic lung disease
    D. LVH
    E. Pleural effusion

8. True statements about MI on the ECG include:
    A. High grade AV block is a possible complication of an acute inferior MI.
    B. ST segment elevation which persists longer than 6 weeks may indicate a ventricular aneurysm.
    C. An acute posterior MI is indicated by loss of R wave in V_2 and V_3.
    D. A Q wave can be normal in V_3.
    E. A Q wave in Lead II is more specific than in Lead III for an inferior MI.

9. True statements about the ST segment and T waves include:
    A. Early repolarization is typically seen in geriatric patients.
    B. A prominent U wave is consistent with hypomagnesemia.
    C. ST segment depression could indicate an acute MI.
    D. Deep T wave inversions in the precordial leads can be seen in patients with subarachnoid hemorrhage.
    E. Upsloping ST segment depression is more specific for ischemia than downsloping ST depression.

10. True statements about the QT interval include:
    A. The QT interval should be less than half of the R-R interval.
    B. Amiodarone can prolong the QT interval.
    C. Hypocalcemia can prolong the QT interval.
    D. Class I antiarrhythmic agents usually shorten the QT interval.
    E. QT prolongation predisposes the patient to ventricular arrhythmias.

11. True statements about medication toxicities and the ECG include:
    A. Accelerated junctional rhythm and atrial tachycardia with AV block are consistent with digoxin toxicity.
    B. Quinidine toxicity produces prolongation of the QRS complex.
    C. Tricyclic antidepressant overdose can produce ST segment depression.
    D. Multifocal PVCs are consistent with digoxin toxicity.
    E. Verapamil overdose can produce profound bradycardia.

12. True statements about the ECG findings in chronic lung disease include:
    A. A prominent negative terminal deflection of the P wave in V_1 is typical.
    B. Right axis deviation is typical.
    C. Tall R waves in V_1 are almost always present.
    D. Low voltage is typical.
    E. An R wave > 12 mm in aVL is typical.

13. True statements about reentrant arrhythmias include:
    A. Reentrant arrhythmias usually start gradually and "warm up" over a period of 10–20 seconds.
    B. Accessory pathways, as in WPW, can participate in reentrant arrhythmias.
    C. Vagal maneuvers are useful in the diagnosis of the supraventricular reentrant arrhythmias.
    D. The commonest cause of reentrant ventricular tachycardia is dilated cardiomyopathy.
    E. Most cases of PSVT involve the AV node.

14. True statements about reentrant arrhythmias include:
    A. Monomorphic PVCs with a fixed coupling interval are consistent with a reentrant mechanism.
    B. One method of treating reentrant arrhythmias involves slowing conduction in one of the reentrant limbs.
    C. IV adenosine frequently terminates atrial flutter.
    D. The ventricular rate in atrial fibrillation increases with exercise.
    E. Atrial flutter usually shows slight variations in the flutter wave rate.

15. True statements about SA conduction abnormalities include:
    A. Second degree SA block Type I can cause group beating of the QRS complexes.
    B. First degree SA block causes PR segment prolongation.
    C. The commonest cause of a pause on an ECG is SA exit block.
    D. Elderly patients with supraventricular tachyarrhythmias can demonstrate a prolonged sinus node recovery time (SNRT).
    E. The sinus node dictates the heart rate because it has the fastest intrinsic rate of depolarization.

16. True statements about atrial fibrillation include:
    A. The commonest cause in the United States is coronary artery disease.
    B. The atrial rate is 400–600.
    C. AV nodal ablation would result in a regular ventricular response.
    D. Atrial fibrillation is a common manifestation of quinidine toxicity.
    E. Usually, only 50 joules of energy is necessary to cardiovert atrial fibrillation.

17. True statements about ectopic arrhythmias include:
    A. Ectopic atrial rhythm and junctional rhythm both have normal P wave axes.
    B. Multifocal atrial tachycardia is usually a consequence of ischemic heart disease.
    C. An ectopic focus is the commonest cause of ventricular tachycardia.
    D. Atrial tachycardia usually has a rate similar to atrial flutter.
    E. Digoxin toxicity should be considered in all cases of ectopic arrhythmias.

18. True statements about ventricular tachycardia include:
    A. Ventricular tachycardia causes AV dissociation by inducing third degree AV block.
    B. Irregular cannon a waves in the neck are consistent with ventricular tachycardia.
    C. Ventricular tachycardia at a rate of 150 is more likely to produce syncope than PSVT with a ventricular rate of 180.
    D. Negative concordance of the QRS complexes across the precordium is consistent with ventricular tachycardia.
    E. The proper treatment for a patient with a wide QRS tachycardia and a systolic blood pressure of 65 mm Hg is immediate cardioversion.

19. True statements about wide QRS tachycardias include:
    A. Intravenous verapamil is extremely useful in differentiating wide QRS tachycardias.
    B. All cases of ventricular tachycardia have AV dissociation.
    C. The longer the QRS duration, the more likely the arrhythmia is to represent ventricular tachycardia.
    D. Ventricular tachycardia requires very high energy levels (eg, 360 joules) to cardiovert.
    E. Ventricular tachycardia is always exquisitely regular.

20. True statements about patients with accessory pathways include:
    A. The presence of a delta wave on the ECG does not exclude the diagnosis of LVH.
    B. Acute infarcts can be detected in patients with WPW on the ECG.
    C. Beta blockers may be useful in the treatment of patients with WPW and PSVT.
    D. WPW can produce a tall R wave in V_1.
    E. Patients with WPW and PSVT in which the direction of current flow is down the accessory pathway and retrograde up the AV node, have a wide QRS tachycardia.

Answers to the Final Examination

The following are correct:

1. B, D, E
2. B, D
3. A, D, E
4. B, C, D
5. C, D
6. A, D, E
7. A, B, C, D
8. A, B, E
9. B, C, D
10. A, B, C, E
11. A, B, C, D, E
12. B, D
13. B, C, E
14. A, B, D
15. A, D, E
16. A, B, C
17. E
18. B, E
19. C
20. B, C, D, E